THE SMART GUIDE TO RHINOPLASTY
WHAT YOU NEED TO KNOW BEFORE GETTING A NOSE JOB

MASOUD SAMAN, MD, FACS

LIMEVI PRESS

Copyright © 2025 by Masoud Saman

All rights reserved. No part of this book may be reproduced or used in any manner without written permission of the copyright owner, except for the use of quotations in a book review.

Published by Limevi Press 240 Central Park South, Suite 2H, New York, NY 10019

ISBN: 979-8-218-63224-3

First Edition 2025

Cover design approved by Lilia, Melodie, and Vianna Saman

Printed in the United States of America

Connect with Dr. Saman on Instagram: @samanplasticsurgery

For information and inquiries, please contact: info@samanmd.com

❀ Created with Vellum

To my mother, whose love, wisdom, and belief in me shaped who I am. You instilled in me a deep appreciation for the arts, the pursuit of knowledge, and the confidence to chase my dreams.

To my late father, a literary man who would have been proud to see this book come to life and to my brother, whose steadfast belief in me never wavered.

To my wife, my rock, my confidante, and my greatest adventure. Your love is my foundation, your support my strength. Your keen eye has made me a better surgeon, but more than that, your presence has made life richer and more beautiful.

To my three little angels, Lilia, Mélodie, and Vianna—you are my heart and my greatest joy. You fill my days with laughter, curiosity, and the kind of love that makes life truly meaningful. Being your daddy is my greatest accomplishment.

To my patients, who trust me with their faces—I do not take it for granted. It is an honor I carry with the utmost care and respect.

And to my teachers—those who have shared their wisdom, challenged me to grow, and even those whose examples showed me a different path—you have all shaped my journey in ways both profound and subtle. I am deeply grateful.

CONTENTS

Foreword — vii
Foreword — xi
Preface — xiii
Part 1: Philosophy and Psychology of Rhinoplasty — xv

1. Introduction — 1
2. My Journey as a Rhinoplasty Surgeon — 6
3. The Importance of the Nose and Its Shape — 16
4. A Brief History of Rhinoplasty — 23
5. Understanding Nasal Anatomy and Ethnic Considerations in Rhinoplasty — 30
6. The Psychology of Rhinoplasty: Understanding the Emotional Factors Behind Surgery — 36
7. Why People Get Rhinoplasty: Motivations and Adaptations — 43
8. Unrealistic Expectations and Body Dysmorphic Disorder (BDD) – When Surgery May Not Be the Right Choice — 49
9. The 80/20 Rule of Aesthetic Surgery — 55
10. Social Media: The Impact of Filters, Influencers, and Online Beauty Standards — 62
11. Breathing Matters: The Functional Side of Rhinoplasty — 67
12. What Is the Best Age for Rhinoplasty? — 73
13. Why Revision Rhinoplasty Is More Complex — 79
Part 2: The Art and Science of Rhinoplasty — 87
14. The Truth About Nonsurgical Rhinoplasty: Illusion, Risks, and the Long-Term Impact — 88
15. The Nose in Facial Harmony: The Art of Balance — 95
16. How to Prepare for Your Rhinoplasty Consultation — 99
17. Computer Simulations and 3D Models — 106

18. Open vs. Closed Rhinoplasty – The Differences, Pros, and Cons — 112
19. Preservation Rhinoplasty vs. Structural Rhinoplasty: an Overview — 119
20. Modern Advances in Rhinoplasty: Technology, Precision, and the Future — 124

Part 3: Making the Right Choice — 129

21. True Craftsmanship and the Pursuit of Excellence — 130
22. Style Matters — 136
23. When Choosing a Rhinoplasty Surgeon — 143
24. How to Assess Before-and-After Photos Critically — 149
25. The Setting Matters as Much as the Surgeon — 153
26. The Financial Aspect of Rhinoplasty: Price, Cost, Value — 158
27. Navigating the Realities of Medical Tourism — 164
28. Common Myths About Rhinoplasty: Separating Fact from Fiction — 172
29. How to Talk to Family and Friends About Your Decision — 178
30. Trusting the Process is Key — 183
31. Final Thoughts — 188

About the Author — 191

FOREWORD

The Smart Guide to Rhinoplasty, written by Dr. Masoud Saman, beautifully answers a fundamental question: What makes a nose "beautiful"?

Rhinoplasty is a unique procedure—one that is not only aesthetic and functional but also deeply technical, artistic, psychological, and social. Changing the nose means changing how one sees themselves. It carries the potential to alter how others perceive us, while also offering an opportunity to improve our relationships with family, friends, and colleagues.

How can the nose represent the center of our personal and social lives? What does it mean for a nose to look natural?

Positioned at the center of the face, the nose inevitably becomes a focal point of communication. While we do not communicate with it directly, it plays a crucial role in our gaze and our smile. In essence, modifying the nose also reshapes our social interactions.

A nose may draw attention due to a flaw, and it is precisely that flaw that rhinoplasty aims to correct. The challenge, however, lies in achieving a result that looks entirely natural. A "natural nose" in terms of communication—with oneself and with others—must meet three essential conditions: it should harmonize with the overall facial structure, eliminate congenital or traumatic imperfections, and avoid surgical flaws that create an artificial "surgical look." When these conditions are met, the nose should go unnoticed after surgery because it blends so seamlessly into the face. This idea aligns with the Japanese concept of *Wasure-Bana*—a nose so natural, it's forgotten.

Why Did Dr. Saman Write This Book?

Dr. Masoud Saman has built an impeccable career, balancing his personal and professional life with remarkable harmony. A tireless worker, he has dedicated himself to mastering facial plastic surgery, particularly rhinoplasty, through rigorous medical and surgical training. His expertise is reflected in his numerous scientific articles, book chapters, presentations, and live surgical demonstrations. He possesses a deep and nuanced understanding of rhinoplasty, which is evident throughout this book. It's no exaggeration to say that I hold great respect for both the man and his work.

Why Is The Smart Guide to Rhinoplasty an Important Book?

This book is accessible, informative, and designed to provide a comprehensive understanding of rhinoplasty for anyone interested. The section on rhinoplasty in adolescents is particularly insightful, and I fully support the approach described in this book. In an era where social media greatly influences self-image, I have no doubt this book will serve as both a scientific and humanistic resource, offering valuable guidance for anyone considering rhinoplasty.

Conclusion

The Smart Guide to Rhinoplasty presents the perspective of a surgeon who strives for excellence in his craft. It not only provides a thorough and objective exploration of rhinoplasty but also addresses patients' concerns—often through real-life testimonials and clinical cases that many readers will find relatable.

Dr. Saman deserves recognition for this outstanding work, which reflects his dedication and commitment to his field. I am honored to have written the foreword to such an exceptional book and extend my sincere gratitude to Dr. Masoud Saman for his remarkable contribution to the field of facial plastic surgery.

Yves Saban, MD

Chairman, European Academy of Facial Plastic Surgery Rhinoplasty Group
Past President, International Rhinoplasty Research Society
Nice, France

FOREWORD

Rhinoplasty is not just a surgical procedure; it is a discipline that demands both technical mastery and an artistic sensibility. The best surgeons in this field are not merely those who learn techniques but those who deeply understand and refine them. Dr. Masoud Saman is one of those rare individuals.

When our paths first crossed years ago, it was immediately clear to me that Masoud Saman was not just another student of surgery—he was an artist, a thinker, and a surgeon who saw beyond the technical steps. In the hands-on training I provided, his ability to grasp the nuances of technique, his attention to detail, and his aesthetic sensibility set him apart. But more importantly, he did not just apply what he learned —he internalized it, evolved it, and made it his own. Today, he stands as not only a highly skilled surgeon but also a leader and an educator in his own right.

This book is a reflection of Masoud Saman's vast experience, refined aesthetic judgment, and dedication to excellence in rhinoplasty. It offers valuable insights not only into the technical aspects of the procedure but also into the philosophy and psychology that underpin it. Whether you are a fellow surgeon seeking to deepen your expertise or a patient looking to understand the journey of rhinoplasty, this book will serve as an essential guide.

Dr. Saman's approach to surgery is thoughtful, patient-centered, and deeply rooted in artistry. Having witnessed his journey firsthand, I have no doubt this book will be an invaluable resource for anyone passionate about rhinoplasty. It is a testament to his commitment, his skill, and his vision for the future of nasal surgery.

Teoman Doğan, M.D., Ph.D.

Plastic Surgeon
Pioneer of Teorhinoplasty: A Minimalist Approach to Rhinoplasty
Istanbul, Türkiye

PREFACE

I've spent years studying, refining, and performing rhinoplasty, but the part of my job that stays with me the most isn't the surgeries—it's the patients. The ones who walk into my office, hopeful, nervous, excited. The ones who come to me after a bad experience, wishing they had known more before making their decision. The ones who have spent years disliking their nose, only to realize that changing it wouldn't fix deeper insecurities. And the ones who, with the right approach and the right expectations, walk away with a result that still feels like *them*—just a version they're happier with.

Rhinoplasty isn't just about changing a nose. It's about understanding what you truly want, why you want it, and what the journey really entails. And yet, in today's world, that understanding is harder to come by than ever. Social media is flooded with before-and-afters, filtered faces, and bold promises. Five-star reviews and glossy websites won't tell you anything about a surgeon's skill, judgment, or whether they're the right fit for *you*. Worse, unrealistic expectations are being sold as reality, making patients chase perfection—something that simply doesn't exist.

I wrote this book because I want you to have what so many patients before you didn't: *the truth*. I want you to know what to look for in a surgeon when all the marketing looks the same. I want you to recognize the red flags. I want you to understand the limitations of surgery, the risks, and the nuances that no one talks about. Most of all, I want you to go into this decision with clarity, not confusion.

This is the book I wish every patient had before stepping into a consultation room. Think of it as your insider's guide—a way to cut through the noise, make informed choices, and, if rhinoplasty is right for you, ensure that your journey is one of empowerment, not regret.

Masoud Saman, MD, FACS

Facial Plastic Surgeon
New York, NY

PART 1: PHILOSOPHY AND PSYCHOLOGY OF RHINOPLASTY

CHAPTER 1
INTRODUCTION

Rhinoplasty is more than just a surgical procedure, it's a journey. For many, it's a deeply personal decision, tied to self-confidence, identity, and even function. Whether you're considering rhinoplasty to enhance your appearance, improve breathing, or correct a previous surgery, making the right choice is crucial. This book is here to help.

After years of intensive training—medical school, a five-year surgical residency in ear, nose, and throat at a top program, and specialized fellowships in head and neck oncology, microvascular reconstruction, skull base surgery, and facial plastic and reconstructive surgery—I earned double board certification in both head and neck surgery and facial plastic surgery. You'd think that after all that, I'd be fully prepared to deliver impeccable results. But in reality, my true education had only just begun. I had just arrived at the base of the mountain.

. . .

In those early years, I focused on imitating what my mentors taught me. I didn't fully understand my own style or how each surgical move affected the final outcome. My results were decent, and my patients were satisfied, but I knew I could do better. I had a vision in my mind for the results I wanted, and what I saw in my post-op photos didn't quite match. I had to strive for improvement.

My wife, a wonderful pediatric dentist with an impeccable eye for detail, has always been my most loving but toughest critic. Her aesthetic judgment is one I deeply respect, and she has an uncanny ability to see what others—including me—might overlook. She never hesitated to gently point out when something in my results could have been better—not to criticize, but to push me. From the perspective of a husband who wanted to impress his wife, this was frustrating to hear at times, but deep down, I knew she was right. And that's when I had a choice: I could either keep doing things the same way and settle for "good enough," or I could push myself to refine, evolve, and elevate my craft. I chose the latter.

I wasn't fully satisfied, so I set out to change that. I had seen masters around the world create extraordinary noses—some had a gift for sculpting the perfect nasal tip, others mastered seamless contours, and some pioneered minimally invasive approaches that left noses looking untouched yet refined. Each had a distinct strength, a unique artistry that translated into exceptional outcomes in a specific aspect of rhinoplasty. So, I sought them out. I shut down my clinic, packed my bags, and traveled across the world to learn from them—one-on-one, in their operating rooms, watching their hands, their choices, their finesse. I studied what made their techniques exceptional, dissected their methods, and absorbed every detail.

Over time, I refined my approach, integrating elements from world-class surgeons while adapting them to align with my personal aesthetic philosophy. What emerged is a technique that reflects my dedication to balance, function, and natural beauty. While every surgeon has their own style, my approach is one I have carefully developed to achieve results that feel both elegant and timeless.

Years later, after countless hours in the OR and continuous refinement of my technique, my wife now looks at my work and gives a nod of approval—well, most of the time. Occasionally, she still raises an eyebrow, and I've come to appreciate that as a reminder that there's always room for growth. Her keen eye keeps me striving for excellence, and for that, I'm grateful.

The truth is, rhinoplasty is not a surgery you can just be *okay* at. It is widely considered the most complex and unforgiving of all aesthetic procedures. The nose is highly intricate—every millimeter matters, every adjustment affects both form and function. A great rhinoplasty requires a full understanding of its structural nuances, the interplay between different components, and how changing one part influences the whole. It's a procedure that demands full focus and true commitment.

Yet, many surgeons don't truly understand the nose—not because they aren't intelligent or well-trained, but because they simply don't do enough rhinoplasties to develop the level of expertise required to master it. If a surgeon performs one rhinoplasty a month while juggling twenty other procedures—facelifts, breast augmentations, liposuction, you name it—they're simply not spending enough time on rhinoplasty. And in surgery, repetition matters.

The more you do, the more you see. The more you see, the more you learn. In my practice, I perform around 200 rhinoplasties per year. That means I don't just operate—I follow 200 unique healing journeys. I see how techniques translate into long-term results, how different patients heal, and how even the smallest refinements can make a difference. I don't rely on static textbook knowledge—I analyze my own work with a critical lens, recognizing patterns, improving strengths, and addressing even rare complications with insight gained from experience. There is power in numbers, and that power is what allows me to keep refining, evolving, and pushing for even better results.

Rhinoplasty requires super-specialization. Sure, there may be, here and there, masters who can do it all (I have yet to meet one), but in my experience and view, to do something really well—at the highest level—a surgeon must be fully committed. It has to be their focus, their passion, their craft.

Unfortunately, misinformation in rhinoplasty is rampant. Many patients come to consultations with expectations shaped by social media—heavily edited photos, unrealistic filters, and misleading trends that make rhinoplasty seem as simple as picking a shape off a menu.

. . .

This book is designed to cut through the noise. We'll cover everything you need to know, from the history of rhinoplasty to modern advances, from the psychology behind nose reshaping to the crucial factors in choosing a surgeon. You'll learn about ethnic considerations, different surgical approaches, and what to expect before and after the procedure. My goal is simple: to empower you with knowledge so that, no matter where you are in your rhinoplasty journey, you can make the best decision for yourself.

Rhinoplasty is not just about changing a nose, it's about balance, harmony, and bringing out the best version of you.

Let's dive in.

CHAPTER 2
MY JOURNEY AS A RHINOPLASTY SURGEON

Ever since I was a child, I wanted to be a physician.

No, I'm kidding. That's not true at all.

No one in my family was a doctor, and I knew little about physicians—except that they intimidated me. As a child, I half-believed they could read my mind—or could they? Later, I saw many as distant, even arrogant. Besides, my family wasn't wealthy. Becoming a doctor felt like a privilege reserved for the well-off—certainly not for someone like me.

I was born into a middle-class family with hardworking parents. My mother juggled clerical jobs to make sure my brother and I never went without—and that we attended the best schools she could afford. She had a deep love for the arts, though she never had the time to fully pursue it. Still, she passed it on to me effortlessly.

I remember sitting with her as a kid, sketching together. I was in awe of how she could bring a rose or a face to life with just a pencil. Even when helping me with school projects, she had a way of turning a plain cardboard collage into something that looked like it belonged in a gallery. Creativity poured out of her.

She found beauty in everything. Music could bring her to tears, architecture left her in awe, and even a simple walk down the street was never just a walk—it was a series of unscheduled stops to admire the way a building's arches framed the sky, how a tree leaned just so, or how the sunlight knew exactly where to land to make the world look like a painting. Her way of seeing things shaped mine. I grew up knowing that art wasn't just something you made—it was something you noticed, something you felt.

Now, in her seventies, she finally has the time to lose herself in that passion. She spends hours in her small art studio, creating—just as I always knew she would. Honestly, I think she's making up for lost time. And judging by the growing piles of canvases, she's got plenty to say.

Unlike many kids in Iranian families, I was never pushed to become a doctor. Honestly, that was probably for the best—because as a child, I was a solid B student, far more interested in soccer and bike rides than anything involving books.

· · ·

But then came fifth grade. I failed an important state-administered math test, and let's just say… it did not go over well at home. My mother, despite the financial strain, hired a private tutor, Mr. Yeganeh, who came to our apartment twice a week to drill me on equations and fractions. At first, I hated every second of it. While my friends played soccer in the street, I was stuck inside reviewing fraction subtractions, wondering if math was some kind of cosmic punishment.

Little by little, something shifted. Studying started to make sense. I went from just getting by to actually excelling. By the time I finished ninth grade at one of Tehran's top schools, I had developed something I never saw coming—a genuine love for learning.

Persians have long had a deep cultural relationship with the nose. Growing up, I remember relatives and family friends discussing rhinoplasty over dinner as casually as if they were debating a new haircut. Who had the best nose job? Who looked *too* done? Who was the hottest rhinoplasty surgeon of the moment? It was practically a national pastime.

I left Iran at fifteen to avoid the obligatory two-year military service I would have been drafted into. My parents were, unsurprisingly, against the idea of sending their teenage son off alone wasn't exactly in their plans. But I fought for it, insisting that staying meant stagnation, that I had no future if I remained. I *needed* to leave. I *had* to make something of myself. Eventually, with heavy hearts, they gave in.

· · ·

I'll never forget my last night in Iran—October 12, 1997. At Mehrabad Airport, as we said our goodbyes, my mother's words stayed with me. She reminded me that while we didn't have much money, she had given me something far more valuable: a foundation for success.

> *"The yearning for excellence—scholastic and artistic—is a kind of wealth,"* she told me. *"Find it within you. Don't waste it."*

As I sat on the bus from the terminal to the airplane, her words echoed in my mind. I promised myself I would make something of my life—without fully knowing what that even meant. I'll spare you the full immigrant saga. Suffice it to say, in America, I worked every job I could find—construction, valet parking, grocery stores, gas stations, and more—to support myself and put myself through school. Then, in 2000, I landed a job as a unit secretary at a hospital in Plano, Texas. It was my first real exposure to healthcare.

Growing up, I saw doctors as authoritative and distant figures. But as I entered the medical field, I met mentors who were generous with their knowledge and guidance, changing my perspective entirely. They invited me into the operating room, shared their experiences, and let me see their world up close. I talked with nurses and patients, listening to their stories, witnessing firsthand how medicine could transform lives.

I was starting to like this field.

One day, after work, I was sitting over coffee with my girlfriend at the time (now my wife), Parya, when I casually said, *"You know, maybe I could become a doctor."* It was the first time I had ever spoken that thought aloud. What followed was one of those long, unforgettable conversations—full of curiosity, big dreams, and the kind of boundless optimism you only have at that age—where you can almost *feel* the course of your life quietly shifting beneath you.

Once the idea took hold, I threw myself into it. I started taking science classes, diving into this new chapter with excitement. Before long, I enrolled in a neuroscience program, determined to take my studies seriously. I still loved the arts, humanities, and languages. So, I took a year off and traveled.

That year was unforgettable. Traveling across France and Spain, busking through cities, wasn't just a way to get by—it was an adventure that made everything feel wide open. Playing on the streets of Paris wasn't just about the music; it was about the energy, the people, and the thrill of figuring things out as I went. Looking back, I think every young person should have a "study abroad" experience, whether it's through school, work, or just throwing themselves into the world. There's nothing like it.

By 2005, refreshed and ready, I began medical school.

Finding My Path in Surgery
At first, I thought I'd become a neurosurgeon—it seemed like the logical next step with my neuroscience background, and let's be honest, it sounded pretty cool. But everything changed one day in medical school when I met a young man born with an untreated cleft lip—simply because he lacked

access to care. Seeing how a facial difference affected not just his appearance but his confidence and emotional well-being was profoundly moving.

Around the same time, I met Dr. Richard Holt, a charismatic facial plastic surgeon whose passion and humanity made an impression on me. Watching him work, I realized *this* was the kind of surgeon I wanted to become. Plus, I found myself deeply fascinated by the intricate anatomy of the head and neck, completely at home in the precision required for facial surgery. That combination of technical skill and life-changing impact was exactly what I had been looking for.

Just like that, my path shifted. I set my sights on facial plastic surgery and never looked back. During medical school, I traveled to Nicaragua and Mexico for mission trips, assisting in pro bono surgeries—something I continue to do to this day. It remains one of the most rewarding parts of my career. In 2006, I was awarded a prestigious National Institutes of Health research grant and moved to Boston to conduct research at Harvard Medical School.

After graduating, I matched into one of the country's most competitive residency programs: Otolaryngology–Head and Neck Surgery at the New York Eye and Ear Infirmary of Mount Sinai. There, I trained in all aspects of ear, nose, and throat surgery, as well as head and neck surgery—including my true passion, facial plastic surgery.

After completing my formal training, I was selected for an advanced fellowship under the American Academy of Facial

Plastic and Reconstructive Surgery, training under Dr. Yadranko Ducic—a surgeon I deeply admire. That year was the most intense of my life. I covered four operating rooms across three hospitals, performing twenty to twenty five surgeries a day: cranial vault reconstructions, oral cancer resections, pediatric cleft repairs, skull base surgeries, and complex reconstructions.

From Dr. Ducic, I learned far more than surgical techniques—I absorbed a philosophy that reshaped my entire approach to medicine. He taught me that true mastery lies in knowing when to push beyond perceived limitations. Beyond skill, he instilled in me something even greater: humility, a respect for the art of surgery, and a deep awareness of the responsibility we hold in our hands.

When I completed my training, he gave me a watch engraved with the words: *"May He always guide your hands."* I still carry that message with me—both on my wrist and in my practice. After that grueling year, he honored me with an unexpected opportunity: an invitation to stay on as faculty, working alongside him to help train the next generation of surgeons.

Just as I was stepping into the professional world, life threw me another incredible twist. On the night my firstborn entered the world, we received a massive bouquet of flowers with a note that simply read:

> *"Dear Dr. Saman, Congratulations on your bundle of joy! We have heard so much about you and would love to discuss a leadership opportunity at our hospital."*

That hospital? The very same one where, years earlier, I had worked as a unit secretary. It was a full-circle moment—one I never could have scripted. On orientation day, as we toured the hospital with the administrators, some of the older nurses even recognized me.

Why I Chose Aesthetic Surgery

I started out in facial plastic surgery with a clear goal: to treat facial abnormalities like cleft lip and palate. But during my training, I found myself drawn more and more to caring for cancer patients. The more tumors I resected, the more frustrated I became with what came next. Sure, we could reconstruct the defect, but too often, the result left patients feeling like strangers in their own skin. They had survived cancer but were still struggling to face the world. Reconstruction alone wasn't enough, it had to be *aesthetic*. It had to restore not just function, but confidence, dignity, and quality of life.

For years, I led one of the largest head and neck oncologic and reconstruction centers in North Texas, treating patients who had lost their faces to cancer or suffered devastating ballistic trauma. It was intense, emotional work—equal parts science and artistry. That experience gave me a uniquely creative, out-of-the-box approach to surgery, one I never would have developed had I trained solely in aesthetics.

I was all in. Our team took on some of the most advanced and challenging cancers—cases others had deemed untreatable. And there were real victories. Patients who had been told there was no hope walked out of the hospital with a second chance. The work was meaningful in the deepest sense—pushing the limits of what was possible, using every skill and resource to fight for lives.

Over time, the weight of it all began to take its toll. It wasn't the long hours or the technical demands—it was the suffering I witnessed day after day. The hard conversations, the battles that couldn't be won, the moments when medicine had nothing left to offer. No matter how much was given, not everyone could be saved. Carrying that reality began to wear me down. I knew I had to make a change.

So, I pivoted. If I was going to focus on facial aesthetic surgery, I wanted to be the absolute best that I could be at it. Some years after completing my formal training, I sought to refine my understanding of both structural and preservation rhinoplasty by learning from leaders in the field. I was fortunate to be among the first surgeons trained in the new wave of dorsal preservation rhinoplasty, and that journey introduced me to two remarkable mentors.

I had the privilege of learning from Dr. Yves Saban, widely regarded as the father of modern preservation rhinoplasty. His meticulous approach and profound understanding of nasal anatomy deepened my appreciation for nasal form and function. In Istanbul, Türkiye, I had the opportunity to learn from Dr. Teoman Doğan, whose refined aesthetic sensibility and systematic, minimalist approach reshaped the way I think about this surgery.

. . .

Beyond the technical side of surgery, what really drives me is an obsession with aesthetics. Good results aren't enough—beauty is about nuance, balance, and proportion. My background in art trained me to notice details others might overlook: the way light and shadow interact on the face, how a nose can complement—or disrupt—the natural flow of someone's features. A well-done rhinoplasty should never announce itself. It should feel effortless, as if the patient was simply born that way.

Teaching and mentorship are integral to my practice. I enjoy exchanging insights with colleagues who visit my practice, as learning is a continuous process for all of us and I must say, I learn just as much from them as they do from me. Every perspective, every question, every discussion pushes me to think deeper and refine my own understanding.

Although growing up I did not know becoming a physician was in the cards for me, life has a funny way of unfolding. My path has been anything but conventional or linear, yet in hindsight, every experience has led me to this moment. And in my heart, I know I'm exactly where I'm meant to be.

Okay, enough about me. Let's talk about rhinoplasty.

CHAPTER 3
THE IMPORTANCE OF THE NOSE AND ITS SHAPE

The human nose is much more than a simple breathing apparatus, it's an anchor of identity, a marker of heritage, and a powerful symbol in language, culture, and history. Its shape and structure have fascinated people for millennia, inspiring everything from mythology to modern beauty ideals. Across civilizations, the nose has been admired, criticized, adorned, exaggerated in art, and even used as a basis for judgment.

Why does this one feature carry so much weight? Why is it so emotionally charged for so many? The answer lies in a mix of evolution, psychology, culture, and history.

The Nose in Self-Perception: Why We See Ourselves Through It

As a facial plastic surgeon, I often meet patients whose concerns about their noses go far beyond aesthetics. Many don't just see their nose as a shape or a size issue but as something that projects an unintended emotion or personality trait.

I've had patients tell me their flaring nostrils make them look constantly angry or that a drooping nasal tip makes them seem sad or tired. Others feel that an overly upturned nose gives them an infantile look, while a convex bridge creates an overly strong or aggressive appearance.

Facial symmetry and balance play a massive role in our self-image, and the nose sits at the center of it all. Unlike the eyes, which are expressive and dynamic, the nose is static yet defining—a feature that cannot be fully concealed with makeup or hairstyling. Because of this, people tend to fixate on it when evaluating their own faces.

In clinical psychology, nasal concerns are one of the most common focuses in body dysmorphic disorder (BDD), further proving how deeply this one feature affects self-esteem.

Why Evolution Shaped Our Noses Differently
We might think of nasal shape as purely an aesthetic variation, but the truth is, our noses evolved for survival. Research from Pennsylvania State University suggests that the diversity in nasal shapes across human populations is directly tied to ancestral climates.

- People whose ancestors lived in cold, dry environments—like Northern Europe—tend to have narrower noses, which help warm and humidify air before it reaches the lungs.
- Meanwhile, populations from hot, humid climates—such as parts of Africa and South Asia—have broader noses, which allow for more efficient air intake.

Genetics also plays a fascinating role. Some studies have traced nasal structure variations back to interbreeding with Neanderthals, influencing the broader nasal structures found in certain populations today. In other words, our noses are not random; they are evolutionary tools once essential for adapting to different environments.

What Makes a Nose Attractive?
Attractiveness is often considered purely subjective, yet deep evolutionary and psychological factors influence why certain nasal shapes are perceived as more desirable.

Symmetry plays a crucial role in perceived beauty, as it signals strong genetic development and minimal exposure to environmental stressors. A nose that is well-proportioned to the rest of the face—whether straight, slightly curved, or subtly upturned—enhances overall facial harmony, creating a balanced and aesthetically pleasing appearance.

Conversely, significant asymmetry or disproportion is often perceived less favorably, as it may, from an evolutionary perspective, suggest developmental irregularities. While beauty standards evolve, the subconscious preference for symmetry and proportion remains a powerful force in shaping our perceptions of attractiveness.

Cultural influences have long shaped perceptions of beauty, including the way we view nasal aesthetics. Throughout history, different societies have idealized different nasal shapes, each carrying its own symbolic meaning.

· · ·

In ancient Greece, the so-called "Greek nose"—a straight, high-bridged profile seen in classical sculptures—was associated with intelligence, nobility, and wisdom. It was a feature celebrated in art and mythology, reinforcing the idea that a strong, well-defined nose signified power and refinement.

During the Renaissance and Victorian eras, beauty standards shifted. In Europe, a small, delicate nose became a marker of aristocratic beauty, associated with refinement and femininity. This preference for petite nasal structures was reflected in paintings, literature, and even social expectations of the time.

Though these ideals have evolved, they continue to shape modern perceptions of beauty. Trends may change, but the cultural weight of historical aesthetics still lingers, influencing how we define balance, proportion, and attractiveness today.

The Nose in Language and Cultural Symbolism

The nose is so central to identity that it has become deeply embedded in language across cultures, symbolizing personality traits and behaviors.

Arrogance is reflected in the phrase *"turning up one's nose,"* while those who meddle are accused of *"sticking their nose where it doesn't belong."* Hard work and perseverance are captured in *"keeping one's nose to the grindstone,"* and a keen sense of intuition is praised as *"having a good nose for things."*

These expressions reveal how the nose, beyond its physical presence, serves as a metaphor for character, perception, and social interaction, shaping the way we describe and understand human nature. Similar idioms exist across cultures. Across cultures and languages, the nose has taken on symbolic meaning, often reflecting personality traits or social perceptions.

In French, a snob is described as having their *nez en l'air*—literally, their nose in the air—suggesting an air of superiority or pretentiousness. In Spanish, boldness and intelligence are sometimes linked to the phrase *tener narices*, which translates to "having noses," implying courage and quick wit.

In Iran, where facial features have long been associated with nobility and character, a high or well-defined nose has been celebrated in Persian poetry and classical art as a symbol of refinement and wisdom. These linguistic expressions reveal how deeply intertwined the nose is with cultural identity, shaping perceptions of status, intellect, and elegance.

The idea that one's social standing could be measured by their nose reflects a broader theme in Persian literature, where physical attributes are deeply tied to personal and moral qualities.

The Nose in Mythology and Literature

Beyond mere function, the nose has long been a storytelling device, transcending language to shape narratives across art, literature, and folklore. The ancient Greeks immortalized gods and warriors in marble, carving strong, defined noses to symbolize power and divinity. This association with strength and identity carried into literature, where the nose often serves as a reflection of character.

Pinocchio's growing nose is a tangible measure of honesty or deception. In *Cyrano de Bergerac*, the protagonist's prominent nose becomes both a testament to his wit and passion and a source of deep insecurity. Villains in folklore and cinema frequently bear exaggerated nasal features—long, crooked, or hooked—visually reinforcing their sinister nature. Disney, in particular, has cemented this trope in the public imagination, portraying witches, evil queens, and greedy characters with sharp, exaggerated noses, while princesses and heroines are consistently drawn with small, delicate features.

Across cultures and centuries, the nose remains more than a feature of the face, it is a symbol, a statement, and a story in itself. Whether intentional or not, these visual cues have reinforced the idea that certain nasal shapes are associated with specific personality traits.

The Nose as a Cultural and Social Marker

Throughout history, the structure of the nose has been deeply intertwined with identity, heritage, and even social status. In ancient Rome, a strong, convex nose was considered a mark of leadership—so much so that emperors and generals were immortalized in statues with this defining feature.

During the European Renaissance, beauty ideals among the aristocracy favored a high, refined nasal bridge, while broader or more prominent noses were unjustly associated with lower social standing. Meanwhile, in parts of the Middle

East and South Asia, a well-defined, prominent nose has long been regarded as a symbol of intelligence, strength, and leadership.

Across cultures and time periods, the nose has carried meaning far beyond its physical function, shaping perceptions of power, beauty, and identity. These shifting ideals highlight how cultural perception often dictates beauty more than biology does.

But no matter the perspective, the nose remains one of the most powerful and defining elements of human appearance —one that has captivated and influenced us for thousands of years.

CHAPTER 4
A BRIEF HISTORY OF RHINOPLASTY

Rhinoplasty, one of the oldest surgical procedures known to humankind, has a fascinating and intricate history that spans thousands of years. It is a procedure that, at its core, has always sought to restore form and function—whether to repair injury, correct congenital defects, or refine aesthetic harmony. Studying the evolution of rhinoplasty is not just an exploration of surgical advancements, but also a reflection of the cultural and societal significance placed on the human nose throughout history.

Ancient Beginnings

The earliest documented evidence of nasal reconstruction can be traced back to ancient India around 600 BCE, where the pioneering surgeon Sushruta described techniques for nasal reconstruction in the *Sushruta Samhita*. At a time when amputation of the nose was a common punishment for crimes or acts of war, the need for nasal reconstruction was pressing. Sushruta developed a method that involved using a forehead flap to rebuild the nose—a technique that although modified and refined, remains foundational in reconstructive surgery today. The intricate measurements and artistic precision detailed in his texts underscore the early recognition that nasal surgery was not merely a mechanical process but an art.

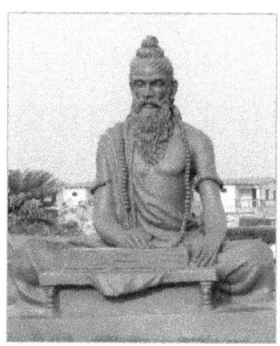

Statue of Sushruta in Patanjali Yogpeeth, Haridwar, India.

Meanwhile, in ancient Egypt, records from the Edwin Smith Papyrus (circa 3000-2500 BCE) provide evidence of nasal fracture treatments, though more in the realm of trauma management than aesthetic reconstruction. In Persia, around the 11th century, the renowned polymath Avicenna documented nasal reconstruction techniques in *The Canon of Medicine*, further demonstrating the procedure's necessity across different civilizations.

The Renaissance of Rhinoplasty in Europe

The practice of rhinoplasty began to make its way into Europe during the Renaissance, in large part due to translations of Arabic medical texts. In the late 16th century, the Italian surgeon Gaspare Tagliacozzi further advanced the field, devising the now-famous "Italian method" that involved using a flap from the upper arm to reconstruct the nose. His book, *Curtorum Chirurgia per Insitionem*, detailed groundbreaking techniques and emphasized the importance of individualizing surgical approaches based on the patient's needs. However, due to religious and societal taboos surrounding bodily alteration, his methods were met with resistance, and interest in nasal surgery waned for some time.

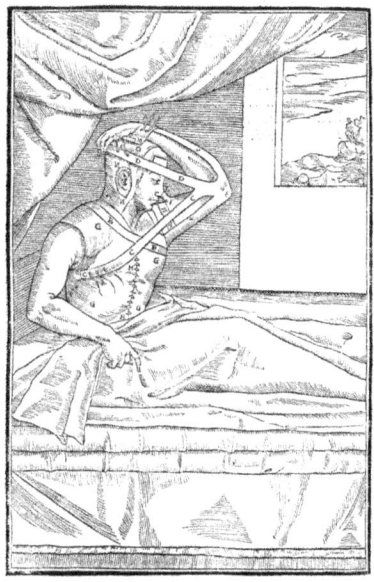

Gaspare Tagliacozzi's 16th-century illustration of the 'Italian method' for nasal reconstruction using a pedicled arm flap.

The 19th and Early 20th Century: The Birth of Modern Rhinoplasty

With the advent of anesthesia and antiseptic techniques in the 19th century, nasal surgery became safer and more approachable. German surgeon Karl Ferdinand von Graefe introduced refinements to the forehead flap technique and coined the term *rhinoplastik* in 1818. Around the same time, Joseph Constantine Carpue performed some of the earliest European nasal reconstructions using the Indian forehead flap method.

. . .

By the late 19th and early 20th centuries, rhinoplasty began transitioning from purely reconstructive to aesthetic procedures. Jacques Joseph, a German orthopedic surgeon, is credited with pioneering modern aesthetic rhinoplasty, developing techniques to reduce nasal humps and refine nasal shape with careful attention to nasal structure and function.

Jacques Joseph's journey to becoming the father of modern aesthetic rhinoplasty was anything but smooth. In fact, when he first presented his work on cosmetic nasal surgery to his surgical peers, he was met with outright ridicule. At a time when surgery was seen as purely functional—meant to repair deformities or save lives—reshaping a nose purely for aesthetics was considered frivolous, even unethical. During one of his earliest presentations, Joseph was reportedly booed off the stage, dismissed by colleagues who saw his work as mere vanity rather than legitimate medicine.

But Joseph was undeterred. He began performing rhinoplasties in secret, working discreetly on patients who sought not just function, but beauty. Many of his earliest clients were wealthy women from Berlin's elite society, as well as actors and performers whose careers depended on their appearance. He also treated young Jewish men who felt their prominent noses made them targets of discrimination in an era of rising antisemitism.

His success grew largely through word of mouth. Patients, thrilled with their transformations, spread his name among high society, and demand for his procedures skyrocketed. Over time, what was once deemed scandalous became accepted, and Joseph was no longer forced to hide his work. He refined techniques that are still the foundation of modern rhinoplasty, including precise cartilage resection, dorsal hump reduction, and the careful preservation of nasal structure to achieve natural-looking results.

Eventually, the medical establishment could no longer ignore his impact. The very peers who once ridiculed him came to recognize Joseph as a visionary, and his techniques were adopted worldwide. Today, his contributions are considered revolutionary, bridging the gap between reconstructive necessity and aesthetic artistry—forever changing the landscape of facial plastic surgery.

The 20th Century and the Refinement of Rhinoplasty

In the early-to-mid 20th century, rhinoplasty underwent significant evolution, leading to greater precision and increasingly natural results. In the United States, John Orlando Roe was among the first to perform closed rhinoplasty, fundamentally changing the field by introducing less invasive nasal reshaping procedures. As the century progressed, influential surgeons like Maurice Cottle and Irving Goldman further refined these methods, combining aesthetic improvements with techniques to address nasal airflow and functional concerns.

The introduction of cartilage grafting during the mid-20th century dramatically transformed rhinoplasty. By utilizing the patient's own cartilage—harvested from the nasal septum, ear, or rib—surgeons could now provide structural support to the nose, ensuring durable, natural-looking results. This advancement was particularly important for patients requiring complex reconstructive or revision surgeries.

Joseph Lothrop notably advanced dorsal preservation rhinoplasty through the development of the "let-down" technique. Maurice Cottle further enhanced these principles with his "push-down" method, allowing surgeons to achieve more natural nasal profiles while preserving the structural integrity of the nasal dorsum. These pioneering contributions form the foundation of modern preservation rhinoplasty, which we'll explore in greater depth in Chapter 19.

More recently, Dr. Yves Saban has been pivotal in revitalizing preservation rhinoplasty through his innovative "high strip" approach. His work has sparked renewed interest in preservation methods, making these techniques increasingly accessible and widely adopted in modern rhinoplasty practice.

Any discussion on contemporary rhinoplasty would be incomplete without recognizing the substantial contributions of Dr. Dean Toriumi. His groundbreaking advancements in structural rhinoplasty have profoundly shaped the field, and his more recent embrace and refinement of preservation rhinoplasty techniques have significantly expanded their application and effectiveness.

Indeed, rhinoplasty as we know it today has been shaped by hundreds—perhaps thousands—of exceptional surgeons who have each contributed in ways both large and small. Giants of the field, such as Samuel Fomon, Jack Sheen, Jack Gunter, and numerous others, have profoundly influenced rhinoplasty practice worldwide. While naming every individual is beyond the scope of this brief history, it is important to acknowledge and express sincere appreciation for the collective impact, dedication, and innovation of these surgeons.

A Personal Reflection on the Evolution of Rhinoplasty

As a facial plastic surgeon, reflecting on rhinoplasty's rich history fills me with humility and gratitude. Each technique I use in my practice today has been shaped by countless surgeons who dedicated their careers to exploration, innovation, and refinement. I have been fortunate to learn from many talented surgeons around the world, integrating time-honored wisdom with modern advancements to help my patients achieve their goals.

While tools and methods continually advance, the essence of rhinoplasty remains constant—a delicate art form that requires precise technical skill and a refined aesthetic eye. Whether restoring function, addressing trauma, or enhancing appearance, rhinoplasty remains one of the most challenging yet rewarding areas of plastic surgery.

CHAPTER 5
UNDERSTANDING NASAL ANATOMY AND ETHNIC CONSIDERATIONS IN RHINOPLASTY

A patient once told me, "I just want a smaller nose." But what does *smaller* truly mean? For one person, it might involve narrowing the tip; for another, reducing the dorsum. Without understanding the fundamental anatomy of the nose, even patients themselves may struggle to articulate exactly what they want or what they genuinely need. In rhinoplasty, an understanding of nasal anatomy isn't reserved only for surgeons; it's essential for anyone contemplating a change to one of the most defining features of their face.

The human nose is profoundly linked to both identity and function. Its shape varies widely across populations, reflecting thousands of years of genetic adaptation, environmental factors, and cultural influences. Effective rhinoplasty requires surgeons to deeply recognize and appreciate these variations—not merely from a technical perspective, but also from aesthetic and anthropological standpoints. Historically, surgical training often focused predominantly on one nasal type, typically the Caucasian nose, causing some surgeons to apply uniform techniques and aesthetic ideals to every patient. This one-size-fits-all approach risks erasing unique ethnic characteristics and frequently leads to unnatural, homogenized outcomes.

Truly successful rhinoplasty is guided by an appreciation for both anatomical precision and aesthetic diversity. By understanding and respecting each patient's unique nasal structure and cultural identity, we ensure outcomes that enhance, rather than erase, individuality.

Basic External Nose Anatomy

To understand rhinoplasty, it's important to be familiar with the external structures of the nose. While every nose is unique, the following terms describe key anatomical landmarks that influence both aesthetics and function.

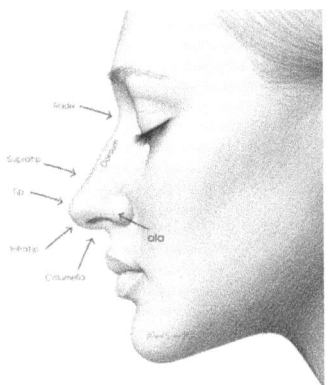

Schematic drawing of the basic external nasal anatomy.

I know this is dry and academic but bear with me. Knowing the "lingo" will help you communicate more effectively with your surgeon.

. . .

Dorsum (Nasal Bridge): The length of the nose from the radix (where the nose starts between the eyes) down to the tip. A straight, convex, or concave dorsum can dramatically affect the profile.

Radix: The uppermost portion of the nose where it meets the forehead. The height of the radix influences how the bridge appears and is an important factor in profile balancing.

Tip: The nasal tip is the most forward part of the nose, where the bridge ends and the nostrils begin. It can vary in shape, projection, and definition. Tip refinement is one of the most intricate aspects of rhinoplasty.

Supratip: The area just above the tip of the nose. A well-contoured supratip transition can make the tip look more refined and natural.

Infratip: The area just below the tip, contributing to how the nose looks from a three-quarter and profile view.

Columella: The tissue separating the nostrils at the base of the nose. Its position and projection impact the appearance of the nasal tip.

Ala (Nasal Wings): The outer edges of the nostrils. Their width, shape, and symmetry play a role in nasal base aesthetics and function.

• • •

Understanding these structures allows both surgeons and patients to better communicate aesthetic goals and understand what changes can be realistically achieved through rhinoplasty.

Nasal Anatomy and Evolutionary Adaptations

Anthropologists classify nasal structures based on the nasal index, which measures the width-to-height ratio of the nose:

Leptorrhine (Narrow): Common in populations from colder, drier climates (e.g., Northern Europeans, some South Asians). Narrow nostrils help humidify and warm the air before it reaches the lungs, which is advantageous in colder environments.

Mesorrhine (Medium-width): Often seen in populations from temperate regions (e.g., Mediterranean, Middle Eastern, Mestizo, some East Asian groups). This nasal type is a balance between function and aesthetics, reflecting mixed environmental adaptations.

Platyrrhine (Broad): Found predominantly in populations from hot, humid regions (e.g., Sub-Saharan Africans, some Southeast Asians, Pacific Islanders). A broader nasal base allows for greater air intake and cooling, an adaptation suited for tropical climates.

These classifications are more than academic—they have real surgical implications. A technique that works for a leptorrhine nose with thin skin and strong cartilage will not work the same way for a platyrrhine nose with weaker cartilage and thicker skin.

Ethnic Variations in Nasal Anatomy

Each ethnic group has distinct nasal characteristics, shaped by evolution, climate, and genetic heritage. These differences must be accounted for in rhinoplasty to maintain harmony with the rest of the face while achieving the patient's aesthetic goals. Although I am not a fan of the term "ethnic rhinoplasty," I am a firm believer that one cannot apply the same set of techniques to all noses. In my practice I operate on a lot patients of Asian or African descent, and believe me, the anatomy if *significantly* different, naturally requiring its own unique skill set for best results.

Preserving Identity vs. Making a Change

Not all patients want to maintain their ethnic nasal characteristics. Some come in specifically requesting a nose that looks different from their natural structure, and that is their choice. Others want subtle refinement while keeping the essence of their nose intact. This is where open discussion is critical. A skilled surgeon must help patients navigate their options while ensuring realistic expectations.

Patients may seek refinement without erasure, improved nasal function, or better profile balance. However, not every request is feasible or advisable. A nose that is too small, too narrow, or excessively upturned on a face with strong, prominent features can create an unnatural, disproportionate look.

• • •

When I Say No as a Surgeon

There are times when a patient brings in a reference photo of a nose that is completely incongruent with their facial features, bone structure, or soft tissue characteristics. While rhinoplasty is a powerful tool, it must be approached with respect for natural anatomy. In these cases, I sometimes have to turn patients away if their expectations are unrealistic or if they are asking for changes that would disrupt the overall balance of their face. This is not about denying patients their autonomy, but rather about guiding them toward decisions that will look natural and harmonious in the long run. A well-done rhinoplasty should look like the nose belongs on that face, not like it was taken from someone else.

CHAPTER 6
THE PSYCHOLOGY OF RHINOPLASTY: UNDERSTANDING THE EMOTIONAL FACTORS BEHIND SURGERY

Rhinoplasty is seldom about aesthetics alone. The nose represents far more than just a physical attribute—it is intricately woven into our identity, culture, personal history, and sometimes even emotional trauma. Positioned centrally on the face, it is the anchor that defines balance and harmony. Often, when patients seek nasal surgery, they aren't simply pursuing cosmetic enhancement; they desire alignment between their inner sense of self and their outward appearance.

The motivations behind choosing rhinoplasty are as diverse as the individuals themselves. Some people have always felt their nose was out of harmony with their other features, while others see nasal surgery as a meaningful step at significant milestones, such as starting college or beginning their careers. Still, there are those who—consciously or subconsciously—hope that transforming their nose will somehow transform their lives, believing it will improve relationships, career opportunities, or overall happiness. When approached with realistic expectations, rhinoplasty can profoundly boost confidence and self-image. However, if the nose becomes a symbol or scapegoat for deeper emotional dissatisfaction, no surgical outcome can fully resolve underlying issues or be considered "good enough."

The Desire for Rhinoplasty Often Begins in Childhood

Many of my patients share a common sentiment: "I've wanted this since I was eleven or twelve years old." Early adolescence is often when we first become deeply aware of how others perceive us. During these formative years, social comparisons become more intense, and for those whose nasal features stand out—due to size, shape, or asymmetry—the nose often becomes a significant source of insecurity.

For some, dissatisfaction arises internally as they notice their nose doesn't align harmoniously with their other facial features. For others, external influences spark their desire for change—a teasing comment from a classmate, an unintended remark from a family member, or simply recognizing they look different from their peers can plant lasting seeds of insecurity.

From a surgical standpoint, rhinoplasty is typically appropriate once facial growth has concluded, generally around age fifteen for girls and sixteen for boys. Many younger patients choose to have surgery ahead of significant life milestones—such as beginning college or starting their careers—to step forward with increased confidence.

• • •

For others, the decision arrives later, often in their mid-twenties to early thirties, once they've gained financial independence and clarity about their aesthetic desires. At this point, they're ready to pursue a goal they've held for years. Likewise, it's not uncommon to see patients in their forties, fifties, and even sixties who, after a lifetime of personal dissatisfaction, finally decide it's time to make a change.

However, not everyone who arrives for a consultation is prepared. Some enter with unrealistic expectations, believing rhinoplasty will resolve issues far beyond aesthetic concerns. Recognizing and managing these expectations is crucial for achieving a genuinely satisfying outcome.

The Lingering Impact of Bullying and Trauma

For some, the desire for rhinoplasty is not just about balance, it is about escaping painful memories associated with their nose. Many patients have vivid recollections of being teased as children, feeling singled out for their appearance.

I once had a patient—let's call her Leila—who had inherited a prominent nasal hump from her father. Her family saw it as a symbol of lineage and pride, but to her classmates, it was something to mock. She was called names like "witch" and "big nose" throughout middle school, and despite her accomplishments and intelligence, she always felt her nose overshadowed everything else about her. At twenty eight, when she finally came in for surgery, she told me: "I don't want to erase my history—I just don't want my nose to be the thing people see first."

• • •

Plastic surgery expert Dr. Mark Constantian has studied the link between childhood trauma and body image dissatisfaction, noting that patients who experience emotional distress in early life are more likely to fixate on physical flaws. For these individuals, rhinoplasty can be a tool for self-empowerment, but it is crucial to understand that it will not erase the past. If deeper emotional wounds are not addressed, no amount of refinement will ever feel like "enough."

When the Nose Becomes a Scapegoat for Life's Problems
While most patients seek rhinoplasty for well-thought-out, reasonable reasons, a subset views their nose as the root of their personal and professional struggles. They believe that if only their nose were different, their entire life would change.

"If I didn't have this hump, I would be more successful."
"If my nose were smaller, I'd be in a happy relationship."
"If my nose were straighter, I wouldn't have been passed over for that promotion."

For these individuals, the nose becomes a scapegoat for deeper dissatisfaction. But when surgery doesn't magically transform their job, relationships, or self-esteem overnight, their focus shifts to minor imperfections in their results.

"Maybe the nose isn't quite straight enough."
"Maybe the tip is still too wide."
"Maybe the nostrils aren't perfectly symmetrical."

This relentless scrutiny can lead to a cycle of dissatisfaction, with patients seeking revision after revision, convinced that the next surgery will finally make everything perfect. But the real issue isn't the nose, it's a deeper psychological struggle that no surgical procedure alone can resolve.

This is why screening for psychological readiness is critical. A good rhinoplasty surgeon must recognize when a patient has unrealistic expectations or is looking for surgery to solve problems it cannot fix. And sometimes, the best thing I can do for a patient is tell them no.

When Rhinoplasty is a Healthy, Positive Decision
The vast majority of my rhinoplasty patients, however, are grounded, well-adjusted individuals who are simply looking to refine their facial harmony. These patients:

- Want to correct a nasal hump, drooping tip, or asymmetry while maintaining a natural look.
- Have realistic expectations—they aren't seeking perfection, just balance.
- Feel confident in most areas of their life but know they would feel better if their nose was in harmony with their face.

These patients are typically the most satisfied with their results because their expectations align with what rhinoplasty can realistically achieve.

Why Rhinoplasty Faces More Resistance Than Other Cosmetic Procedures
One of the most fascinating aspects of rhinoplasty is the resistance patients face from those around them. When someone gets braces for crooked teeth, no one questions the

decision. But when someone wants to straighten a crooked nose, they are often met with:

"You should love yourself the way you are."
"That's your grandfather's nose—you should keep it."
"You don't need to change yourself."

This speaks to how closely the nose is tied to identity. While teeth are seen as functional, the nose is regarded as a defining familial or ethnic trait. Altering it is sometimes perceived—not just by family, but by broader society—as an erasure of heritage, even when that's not the patient's intention at all.

Conclusion: The Balance Between Psychology and Surgery

Rhinoplasty is never just about changing a nose, it's about helping people feel like the best version of themselves. But it cannot and should not be expected to fix deeper emotional wounds.

A well-performed rhinoplasty should never erase identity, it should refine, enhance, and bring harmony to the face without making the nose its defining feature. When approached with a healthy mindset and realistic expectations, rhinoplasty can be a deeply rewarding, confidence-enhancing journey.

And as a surgeon, there is no greater satisfaction than seeing a patient finally feel at peace with their reflection—not because they've "fixed" something, but because they finally feel that what they see in the mirror matches who they truly are. Self-acceptance and cosmetic surgery are not mutually exclusive.

In the next chapter we will explore some more common reasons and motivations behind why individuals may seek a rhinoplasty.

CHAPTER 7
WHY PEOPLE GET RHINOPLASTY: MOTIVATIONS AND ADAPTATIONS

"It Just Doesn't Fit My Face"

Have you ever looked in the mirror and felt like your nose just doesn't belong? Not bad—just...off? That's something I hear often from my patients. They don't necessarily want a smaller nose or a completely different one. They want a nose that looks like it was meant for them.

Sometimes, the imbalance is subtle—a small, delicate face with a dominant nose, or a soft, feminine jawline contrasted by a sharp, angular bridge. Other times, it's more dynamic, something they only notice in motion. One of the most common complaints I hear isn't about how the nose looks at rest, but what happens when they smile.

Many patients tell me they avoid big smiles in photos because they feel their nose takes over their entire face. As they smile, the tip drops, the nostrils flare, and suddenly, all they notice is their widening nose. Some even train themselves to smile minimally or keep their lips pressed together, afraid that a full expression will make their nose look exaggerated. But this comes at a cost. Smiling is a social cue, and when someone holds back, others may misinterpret them as cold, unapproachable, or sad. In reality, they're not unhappy, they're just self-conscious.

These patients aren't asking for a dramatically different nose. They simply want a nose that fits their face no matter what it's doing—whether they're laughing, talking, or caught mid-expression in a candid photo.

When Puberty Changes Everything

For some, the biggest shock of adolescence wasn't their growth spurt, it was their nose changing seemingly overnight. The once small, delicate nose they had as a child suddenly grew into something unrecognizable. A dorsal hump appeared out of nowhere. The tip became bulbous or started drooping. While the rest of their face stayed soft and youthful, the nose took on a life of its own.

Many patients tell me they used to love their childhood nose. They didn't think about it until puberty reshaped it into something that felt foreign. In these cases, they're not looking for a "new" nose; they just want to restore the face they feel they lost.

When Teasing Becomes a Mirror

Most people don't analyze their own features until someone else points them out. Many of my patients remember the exact moment they became self-conscious about their nose—often around nine or ten years old, when schoolyard teasing begins.

One patient told me, *"I never thought about my nose until a boy in fifth grade called me 'toucan.'"* Another said, *"The kids in middle school used to call me 'witch' because of my profile."*

For some, the teasing was lighthearted and brushed off. For others, it was relentless, leaving scars far deeper than just the shape of their nose.

I remember a teenage patient—I'll call her Emily—who had been painfully self-conscious about her nose for years. As we spoke during her consultation, she hesitated before admitting, *"I've spent most of my life trying to hide my profile."* She told me how, in school, she would always sit with her back against the wall so no one could see her from the side. In class, she kept her head down, pretending to be focused on her work, not because she wasn't engaged but because she couldn't bear the thought of someone whispering about her nose.

When I asked her why she wanted rhinoplasty, she didn't mention beauty. She didn't say she wanted to look a certain way. She just said, *"So I can finally look people in the eye."*

For patients like Emily, rhinoplasty isn't about vanity. It's about relief.

Small Tricks to Shift Attention

People are incredibly resourceful when it comes to adapting to features they feel self-conscious about. Some subtly adjust their eyebrows—plucking or filling them in differently—to create the illusion of balance. Others always tilt their head in photos, knowing exactly which angle makes their nose look straighter or more refined. Hairstyles become another tool, with bangs or layers strategically placed to frame the face and direct attention elsewhere.

Jewelry plays a similar role. A well-placed nose ring, stud, or septum piercing can act as a focal point, pulling attention toward the jewelry rather than the bridge or tip of the nose. Someone with a prominent dorsal hump may wear a nose ring to subtly shift focus to the side of their nose, while a small stud can create an impression of refinement. Some patients don't even realize why they gravitate toward certain piercings—it just feels right to them.

Glasses are another quiet trick. Bold, oversized frames cover much of the nasal dorsum, softening or even concealing features like a hump or asymmetry. The contrast between large glasses and facial features can create an illusion of proportion, making the nose seem smaller in comparison. Some patients tell me they feel like a different person with glasses on, as if they're able to hide behind them. After rhinoplasty, they often find they no longer feel the need to wear statement frames because, for the first time, they feel comfortable letting their nose be fully seen.

When Trauma Changes Everything

Not everyone seeking rhinoplasty has had the same nose

their entire life. Some had a nose they loved until an injury changed it.

I see many patients whose noses were altered by sports injuries, car accidents, childhood falls, or even unnoticed trauma. Some people don't even realize they broke their nose until years later, when they look at old photos and notice how different their profile used to be. For these patients, rhinoplasty is less about changing their nose and more about getting it back—restoring what once felt like *them* and improving function, particularly if breathing was affected.

When the Nose Carries Emotional Weight

For some, a nose isn't just a facial feature, it's a painful reminder of the past. I have treated patients who sought rhinoplasty not for aesthetics, but to distance themselves from a part of their identity they wanted to leave behind.

One patient told me, *"Every time I look in the mirror, I see him."* Another said, *"I feel like I can't escape my past."* These were patients whose noses bore an undeniable resemblance to an abusive parent.

These cases are deeply personal. The surgery is not about vanity; it's about reclaiming identity, breaking free from something painful, and looking in the mirror without feeling haunted.

The Wedding Effect and Other Milestones

A wedding is one of those once-in-a-lifetime moments

where people want to feel their absolute best, knowing their face will be captured in pictures that will last forever.

I had a patient, Sophia, who was thrilled to be getting married. But when she scrolled through her engagement pictures, her heart sank. She hadn't realized how much she disliked her profile until that moment. *"I never thought I needed a nose job,"* she told me, *"but now I can't unsee it."*

She struggled with whether it was vain to have surgery for a big event. The more we talked, the more she realized it wasn't just about the wedding. She wasn't changing her nose for one day, she was making a change for every day after.

It's not just weddings. People come to me before major milestones—important career shifts, public speaking engagements, reunions, and other defining moments where they want to feel confident, knowing all eyes (and cameras) will be on them.

A good rhinoplasty should enhance confidence and self-acceptance, not fuel an endless cycle of dissatisfaction. As a surgeon, my role isn't just to operate, it's to listen, to guide, and, when necessary, to protect patients from making a decision that won't serve them.

CHAPTER 8
UNREALISTIC EXPECTATIONS AND BODY DYSMORPHIC DISORDER (BDD) – WHEN SURGERY MAY NOT BE THE RIGHT CHOICE

A young woman once sat across from me in my office, clutching a photo of herself—except it wasn't really her. The image had been edited beyond recognition. "I want my nose to look like this," she said, her voice filled with both hope and desperation. But what she was chasing wasn't a nose—it was an illusion. And illusions can't be surgically created.

Rhinoplasty is a powerful tool. It can refine features, correct functional issues, and, in the right circumstances, significantly improve a person's self-confidence. Like any tool, its success depends on how and why it is used. Not every person seeking a rhinoplasty is an ideal candidate. Some come in with realistic goals and a clear understanding of what surgery can and cannot achieve. Others, however, arrive with expectations that no surgeon, no matter how skilled, can fulfill.

I have had patients bring in heavily edited or filtered images, aspiring to an aesthetic that does not align with their anatomy or, in some cases, with reality itself. This is where the conversation shifts from surgical technique to psychology.

The Problem with Perfection
One of the greatest misconceptions about rhinoplasty is the belief that a perfect nose exists. It doesn't.

Even the most famous, admired noses—those gracing the faces of Hollywood stars or social media influencers—aren't perfect in real life. They are well-lit, well-angled, and, more often than not, digitally enhanced. Patients sometimes bring in these images, convinced that perfection is attainable. But perfection is not the goal, harmony is. A nose should look like it belongs on your face, not someone else's.

Patients with unrealistic expectations often believe that changing their nose will fix other aspects of their life—relationships, career success, or general happiness. While a rhinoplasty can certainly boost confidence, it is not a cure-all for deeper insecurities or unhappiness. When I sense that a patient may be expecting surgery to solve non-physical issues, I take a step back. If surgery is being sought for the wrong reasons, it's often a sign that it should not be pursued at all.

Understanding Body Dysmorphic Disorder (BDD)
Body Dysmorphic Disorder (BDD) is not simply being self-conscious, it's an all-consuming obsession with a perceived flaw, often one that others don't even notice.

· · ·

In the context of rhinoplasty, BDD can manifest as extreme dissatisfaction with the nose, despite an objectively normal or even aesthetically pleasing structure. Patients with BDD often take endless selfies from different angles, trying to analyze every tiny detail. They may fixate on mirrors or avoid them altogether. Some feel distressed even after multiple surgeries, constantly seeking "one more fix." The problem isn't the nose, it's how they see it.

A patient who is obsessive in their analysis of their nose may not be the best candidate for surgery. When I meet with patients, I always encourage them to take a moment to look inward. How do they handle imperfections in other areas of life? Are they the type of person who can appreciate progress, or do they fixate on what's still missing? Do they tend to see the glass as half full or half empty? Most importantly, will they find satisfaction in the significant improvements we achieve, or will they become consumed by the tiny, unchangeable details? These are the kinds of questions that help determine whether rhinoplasty will bring genuine confidence or just fuel an endless cycle of dissatisfaction.

As a younger surgeon, I sometimes missed the warning signs of BDD or felt pressured into taking on cases—sometimes manipulated into it, other times overcome with sympathy. Every time, I regretted it. The outcome was never truly satisfying for either the patient or me. Now, with experience (meaning I have made mistakes and learned from them), I am very clear with my patients. A consultation is not a promise that surgery will be performed, nor is surgery a guarantee of a specific aesthetic outcome. Instead, our goal is improvement in the aesthetic direction we agree upon together.

· · ·

When I Say No and Why Some Patients Don't Take it Well
There are times when the best decision I can make as a surgeon is to say no.

While some surgeons might operate on anyone willing to pay, I take a different approach. Performing a surgery that will not bring true satisfaction—whether due to unrealistic expectations, psychological concerns, or an obsession with perfection—is a disservice to both the patient and the profession.

Sometimes, patients leave upset because I refuse surgery. I have even had frustrated patients leave negative reviews online, as if denying them surgery was an injustice. "How dare he turn me down?" some might write. I would rather deal with their frustration upfront than perform a surgery that leaves us both disappointed.

I remember a patient who had already undergone two rhinoplasties and still wasn't happy. She wanted me to operate again, convinced that this time, she would finally be satisfied. As we spoke, I realized she wasn't seeking refinement, she was seeking relief from an internal struggle that surgery could never fix.

I told her gently, "I don't think surgery is the right path for you." She left frustrated. But months later, she emailed me.

"Thank you. I didn't want to hear it then, but I realize now that I was chasing something that surgery couldn't fix. I started therapy, and for the first time, I'm learning to see myself differently—not just through the lens of my nose, but through the lens of self-acceptance."

That email confirmed what I already knew—sometimes the best decision is to say no.

How I Assess Expectations
During consultations, I take the time to ask patients key questions to better understand their motivations. What specifically bothers them about their nose? What kind of changes are they hoping for? Beyond aesthetics, what do they believe this surgery will bring to their lives? I also want to understand how much space these concerns occupy in their minds —do they think about their nose occasionally, or is it a daily preoccupation? If they've had previous surgeries, were they satisfied with the results, or are they still searching for something they can't quite define?

The way a patient answers these questions tells me a lot. If their expectations seem unrealistic or if they show signs of obsessive thinking, I take extra care in explaining what rhinoplasty can and cannot do. Sometimes, the best thing I can do as a surgeon is to gently suggest that surgery may not be in their best interest. It's not always what patients want to hear, but in many cases, it's exactly what they need to hear.

Final Thoughts: The Art of Knowing When Surgery Isn't the Answer
A responsible rhinoplasty surgeon does more than sculpt noses, they guide patients toward choices that will genuinely

benefit them. Sometimes, that means advising against surgery altogether. And that, in itself, is part of the art of rhinoplasty.

If you're considering rhinoplasty, take a moment to reflect on your motivations. Are you seeking a natural, harmonious enhancement, or are you chasing an unattainable idea of perfection? Will you appreciate meaningful improvement, or will you fixate on every small imperfection?

The right surgeon will help you find clarity. If they tell you surgery might not be the right choice for you, trust that their advice comes from experience and is given in your best interest.

In the next chapter, we will explore a related concept—the 80/20 rule—and take a deeper look at how expectations and personal perspective shape the way we see outcomes.

Rhinoplasty should not be about chasing an illusion of flawlessness. It should be about refining what is already there, enhancing confidence, and respecting one's natural beauty. The best results don't just bring aesthetic change—they bring peace of mind.

CHAPTER 9
THE 80/20 RULE OF AESTHETIC SURGERY

Sofia stood in front of the mirror, her fingers tracing the bridge of her nose. Her expression was unreadable at first, but then she whispered the words I had heard so many times before.

"I hate it."

I watched her closely. The nose reflected back at her was exactly what we had planned—balanced, refined, elegant. The dorsal hump was gone. The tip was softened. It fit effortlessly with the rest of her face, no longer a separate feature demanding attention. But none of that mattered.

She didn't see what was there. She saw what wasn't.

"There's a shadow here," she said, pointing to an area so subtle I had to lean in to even register it. Her eyes darted between

angles, dissecting every detail, searching for something—some imperfection, some evidence that the result wasn't perfect. I had seen this before.

The 80/20 Rule of Surgery

The first time I heard about the 80/20 rule in plastic surgery, it was from a surgeon I deeply respect, Dr. Mike Nayak. His words stuck with me:

"No surgery gets a patient 100% of the way to their ideal result. At best, we get them to 80%. The remaining 20%? That's life."

That doesn't mean surgery isn't worthwhile. It doesn't mean we don't strive for the 100%. It certainly doesn't mean we don't give our 100%. It just means that achieving a 100% result is not possible.

That 80% can be life-changing. It can boost confidence, restore harmony, and help someone finally feel at peace in their own skin. But there will always be a fraction left untouched—some minor asymmetry, an imperfection only the patient will notice, a lingering expectation that reality could never quite match.

It's human nature to focus on the small things. Years ago, when my wife and I bought our first home, the walls of the children's rooms were covered in crayon drawings and tiny handprints. When the painters finished, I stepped back, admiring the fresh, pristine walls.

. . .

My wife, on the other hand, walked in, took a careful look around, and immediately noticed a single drop of paint on the doorframe. It wasn't that she didn't appreciate the transformation—she did—but her eye naturally went to the one thing that was out of place. Same room; different perspectives.

Surgery is much the same. As surgeons, we strive for precision, but absolute precision is only half of the equation. The other half is how the body heals—something we cannot fully control. Factors like skin thickness, cartilage strength, and individual healing responses all play a role in the final outcome. No matter how meticulous the surgical execution, healing is unpredictable. I try to explain this to patients, but sometimes humor makes the point better. I joke that in surgery, I can be as precise as a master sculptor, but once healing begins, Mother Nature takes over and she doesn't always take requests.

The Myth of Perfection

The idea that surgery can create a "perfect" result is seductive. With modern technology, precision tools, and years of expertise, many patients assume we can sculpt a nose exactly to their vision—flawless from every angle, symmetrical under every light.

But nature doesn't work that way. Even in the best-case scenario, when healing goes smoothly and every technical detail is executed flawlessly, the maximum improvement is about 80%. The remaining 20% is beyond our control—anatomic limitations, how tissue settles, how time reshapes the final outcome.

· · ·

For a first-time rhinoplasty, the goal is 80/20. For revision rhinoplasty, it's more like 70/30—or even 60/40. These aren't hard numbers; they're a way of framing reality.

The 70/30 Reality of Revision Surgery

Revision rhinoplasty presents a unique set of challenges. Scar tissue from previous surgeries can obscure anatomical landmarks, making dissection more complex. The structural integrity of the nose may be compromised, requiring cartilage grafts from the ear or rib. Healing patterns become even more unpredictable.

Patients who have already experienced disappointment with a prior surgery often develop heightened sensitivity to even minor imperfections. Their trust in the process has been shaken, and they naturally scrutinize every detail with a mix of hope and fear. Some eventually relax into the healing process, seeing the positive changes over time. Others, however, struggle to shift their focus from small flaws, making it difficult to appreciate the overall improvement.

Revision surgery is not about erasing the past, it's about making the best of what remains. It's not a fresh start. It's a rescue mission.

At some point, healing becomes about acceptance, about recognizing when to step back and appreciate the progress rather than fixating on the imperfections. There is a quiet wisdom in knowing when to let go, in understanding that chasing perfection will only lead to frustration. The goal is not to erase, but to enhance—to refine, to balance, to bring harmony to what already exists.

The Beauty in Imperfection

In Japanese culture, there is a philosophy known as *wabi-sabi*—the appreciation of imperfection, the beauty in things that are slightly flawed.

There is an ancient practice called *kintsugi*, where broken pottery is repaired with gold lacquer. The cracks are not hidden; they are highlighted, transformed into something unique and beautiful.

Surgery should be viewed in the same way. If we attempt to erase every perceived flaw, we risk erasing identity. If we chase perfection, we chase something that doesn't exist. But if we learn to appreciate transformation rather than fixate on what remains, we find peace in the process.

Sofia couldn't see her gold lacquer yet. She was still searching for cracks.

Are You Ready for Surgery?

This is why I always ask my patients: Are you seeking improvement, or are you chasing an unattainable ideal? Can you embrace change, or will you fixate on the details? Are you mentally prepared for the healing process, which is just as important as the surgery itself?

. . .

The happiest patients are the ones who step back and take in the whole picture. The most frustrated are those who zoom in on imperfections no one else notices. What you choose to focus on will define your experience.

Surgery is a Process, Not a Moment

Surgery doesn't end the moment you wake up from anesthesia. It unfolds over weeks, months, sometimes a full year. The nose you see at one-month post-op is not your final nose. Swelling will shift, contours will refine, small irregularities will smooth out.

This is why mindset is just as important as the surgeon's skill. If you can embrace the 80/20 rule, trust the process, and accept that your result will be beautiful but not mathematically perfect, you will be a much happier, more satisfied patient.

If that remaining 20% will consume you—if you'll spend your days staring into a magnified mirror, analyzing every shadow, comparing yourself to filtered images—then perhaps surgery isn't the right choice. The goal is not flawlessness. The goal is balance, confidence, and harmony.

Seeing the Whole Picture

Months later, Sofia returned for a follow-up. This time, she wasn't searching for flaws. She wasn't analyzing angles in the mirror. She wasn't dissecting the details.

• • •

She smiled. *"You know what's funny?"* she said. *"Now when I look at my face, I don't see my nose. I just see... me."*

In that moment, I knew she was finally seeing what I had seen all along.

CHAPTER 10
SOCIAL MEDIA: THE IMPACT OF FILTERS, INFLUENCERS, AND ONLINE BEAUTY STANDARDS

A Double-Edged Sword
A nineteen-year-old patient sat in front of me, clutching her phone. "This is what I want," she said, turning the screen toward me. On it was an AI-generated version of her face, her nose altered into something that didn't exist in nature. I sighed. I had seen this before—many times.

Social media has completely reshaped the way people perceive beauty. Instagram, TikTok, and Snapchat have given patients unprecedented access to before-and-after results, surgical techniques, and firsthand accounts of rhinoplasty. With this exposure comes a cost—unrealistic expectations, distorted beauty ideals, and the pressure to conform to a curated version of reality.

The Illusion of Perfection
I live in NYC. I literally walk past thousands of faces every week—beautiful faces by human standards, not by

some fake, unattainable social media filter standard. Yet, many people have lost grip on what natural beauty even looks like. I treat models, influencers, and celebrities, and I see them without makeup or filters. Many don't look anything like their profile photos. This illusion of perfection—of flawless skin, perfect symmetry, and "perfect tens"—is just that: an illusion. A carefully curated selection of photos and videos, captured in the best lighting and angles, portraying an effortless, glamorous life.

It saddens me that our youth—and even many mature individuals—are now living under these impossible beauty standards and pressures. No wonder youth depression has skyrocketed. We're losing our sense of what normal beauty is. The objective and the subjective are diverging too much.

To show this, I started a photographic art project called **Face x Face NYC** (said "Face by Face"). We take standardized photographs of thousands of individuals in NYC from all walks of life—same lighting, same zoom, same lens, same settings—to reveal a simple truth: every single face is *perfectly imperfect*. No filters, no distortions, just real, human beauty. This is a work in progress, but it's coming along.

The Good: Transparency, Access, and Global Collaboration

Social media has removed traditional barriers between patients and surgeons. In the past, people relied on word-of-mouth or office albums with limited before-and-after photos. Now, they can scroll through hundreds of rhinoplasty results, compare techniques, and evaluate a surgeon's work in real time. This has made patients more informed than ever.

· · ·

For surgeons, social media has pushed us to refine our craft. We no longer work in isolation—we exchange insights with specialists worldwide, discuss complex cases, and educate the public on procedures and recovery. It has also helped demystify surgery, breaking down myths and misinformation.

The Bad: Unrealistic Beauty Standards and Self-Perception
But there's a darker side. Social media has created an obsession with an impossible standard of beauty. Filters, digital editing, and AI-generated images have made people chase a look that isn't real.

At least a few times a week, I have patients bring in heavily edited photos, asking for a nose that is physically impossible. Some compare their healing process to someone else's Instagram journey, forgetting that every face is unique and recovery is unpredictable. Even selfies are misleading—front-facing cameras can distort proportions, making noses appear 30% larger than they actually are. This has fueled a rise in *selfie dysmorphia*, where people fixate on a distorted version of themselves.

The Hidden Cost: Social Media and Mental Health
Beyond aesthetics, social media has had a profound impact on self-esteem, particularly among younger patients. I see it firsthand.

Some patients, barely out of their teens, don't actually dislike their nose—they've just been ridiculed for it online. The comments can be cruel, and no one should feel "less than" because of an arbitrary digital standard.

. . .

The comparison trap is one of the biggest psychological challenges of this generation. Social media makes people believe they need to look flawless from every angle, all the time, as if they live inside a filter. This obsession has fueled a rise in body dysmorphia and an intolerance for natural variations in facial features.

The Illusion of Effortless Beauty

Another major issue is how social media distorts the perception of recovery. Influencers document their rhinoplasty journeys, but rarely show the full, raw healing process. Instead, they post curated content that makes recovery seem effortless.

Patients see these polished images and expect swelling to disappear overnight, bruising to be minimal, and results to be instant. But rhinoplasty takes time. Healing is gradual. There is no instant filter effect. Some surgeons contribute to these false perceptions by using different lenses, lighting, and even makeup in post-op photos to enhance results. This misleads patients and sets up unrealistic expectations.

When Medicine Becomes a Performance

Social media hasn't just changed how patients perceive beauty, it has also changed how some surgeons present themselves.

There is a growing trend of surgeons prioritizing personal branding over patient care, chasing virality with dramatic hooks and misleading content. Some push surgical trends over long-term aesthetics, while others use work that isn't even theirs to gain followers. Worse, some practices treat rhinoplasty like a retail product—offering flash sales and discounts, commodifying surgery as if it were a handbag or a pair of shoes.

The rise of patient-influencers has further blurred ethical lines. Many are financially incentivized to endorse certain surgeons or procedures, turning what should be genuine experiences into paid marketing.

If we're not careful, we risk losing sight of why we entered this profession in the first place. Aesthetic surgery isn't about fame, likes, or engagement. It's about helping people. The moment we let social media dictate our ethics, we don't just lose credibility—we jeopardize the integrity of our field.

The Social Media Paradox

Social media is neither inherently good nor bad—it's a tool, and its impact depends on how it's used. It has empowered patients, connected surgeons, and brought aesthetic medicine into the mainstream. It has also fueled unrealistic ideals, misleading narratives, and an unhealthy obsession with perfection.

Rhinoplasty isn't about chasing trends or fitting into a viral mold. It's about refining features while preserving identity. No filter, no algorithm, and no viral post should have the power to dictate a person's self-worth.

CHAPTER 11
BREATHING MATTERS: THE FUNCTIONAL SIDE OF RHINOPLASTY

When you look at a nose, what do you notice first? Its shape? Symmetry? How well it fits a person's face? Aesthetics are usually what draw attention, but the most important function of the nose isn't how it looks—it's how it breathes.

Nasal breathing is something most people take for granted—until they can't. Many patients come in seeking rhinoplasty to improve the appearance of their nose, only to discover afterward just how much nasal function impacts their quality of life. Some even break down in tears, not because of how their nose looks, but because they've never been able to breathe this well in their entire lives.

A well-performed rhinoplasty doesn't just refine the external shape of the nose; it should also preserve—or even enhance—airflow. When breathing is optimized, patients often experience unexpected benefits: deeper sleep, better exercise performance, improved energy levels, and even reduced snoring.

. . .

For some patients, airway issues are the main reason they seek surgery. A deviated septum, nasal valve collapse, or chronically enlarged turbinates can make breathing difficult, leading to fatigue, mouth breathing, poor sleep quality, and difficulty with physical activity. Others may have never struggled with nasal obstruction before surgery but develop breathing issues if rhinoplasty is performed without careful attention to airway mechanics.

Understanding the balance between form and function is what separates aesthetic rhinoplasty from truly great rhinoplasty. A nose that looks perfect but doesn't breathe properly is not a success.

More Than Just a Nose Job: My Journey from Reconstruction to Aesthetics

Before I dedicated my practice entirely to facial aesthetics, my work was rooted in nasal and sinus reconstruction. As the Director of Facial Reconstruction at a major metropolitan trauma hospital, I treated some of the most complex nasal cases—patients who had lost their noses due to trauma, cancer, or congenital conditions. These cases weren't about subtle refinements; they were about rebuilding noses from scratch while maintaining or restoring function.

I worked with techniques like rib cartilage grafting, forehead tissue flaps, and microvascular free flaps, all of which required meticulous planning to ensure that breathing wasn't compromised in the process. These experiences taught me an important lesson: the nose isn't just a feature of the face, it's a vital part of how we breathe, sleep, and function.

When I transitioned into aesthetic rhinoplasty, I carried this philosophy with me. Every rhinoplasty I perform is guided by the principle that function and aesthetics must always coexist. The idea that cosmetic and functional nasal surgery are separate is a misconception. A rhinoplasty that prioritizes aesthetics at the expense of breathing is incomplete. And a surgery that improves function but ignores aesthetics may not align with a patient's goals.

This perspective shapes every rhinoplasty I do. I'm not just thinking about how a nose will look in photos—I'm thinking about how it will function for the next twenty, thirty, or forty years.

The Life-Changing Benefits of Better Breathing
When nasal function is restored, the improvements go beyond just feeling "less congested." Breathing properly through the nose impacts multiple areas of health:

- **Better Sleep & Less Snoring** – Many patients experience deeper, more restful sleep after nasal airway surgery, as improved nasal breathing regulates oxygen levels and airflow.
- **Improved Athletic Performance** – Optimal nasal breathing boosts endurance, reduces fatigue, and enhances oxygen delivery, helping patients feel less winded and perform better during exercise.

- **Less Mouth Breathing & Dryness** – Fixing nasal obstruction restores natural breathing, reducing dry throat, bad breath, and dental issues.
- **Sharper Focus & Mental Clarity** – Better oxygen intake improves brain function, reducing brain fog and increasing energy and concentration.

Some patients have spent their entire lives thinking that "this is just how I breathe", unaware that their chronic congestion, snoring, or poor sleep quality was due to an anatomical issue. The moment their nasal passages open up—sometimes for the first time ever—it can be an emotional, even life-changing experience.

How the Nose Regulates Breathing

Breathing through the nose is much more than simply pulling in air, it's a sophisticated system that filters, regulates, and optimizes each breath. The nose plays a crucial role in overall health by warming and humidifying the air before it reaches the lungs, preventing irritation. It also acts as a natural purifier, filtering out dust, allergens, and pollutants, while regulating airflow resistance to ensure efficient oxygen exchange.

For air to move freely, it must pass through three key anatomical areas. The nasal valves, the narrowest part of the airway, control airflow resistance. If these structures weaken or collapse inward, breathing becomes restricted. The septum, the central cartilage and bone that separate the nostrils, can become deviated, leading to chronic congestion and obstructed airflow on one or both sides. Inside the nose, the turbinates help regulate and humidify air, but when they become enlarged due to allergies, chronic inflammation, or structural issues, they can block nasal breathing entirely.

A well-planned rhinoplasty should take all these factors into account, ensuring that any refinements not only enhance the nose's appearance but also improve long-term airflow and function.

Why Rhinoplasty Can Improve Breathing

While many people associate rhinoplasty purely with cosmetic goals, it can be a powerful tool for improving nasal function when performed with the right expertise.

What Rhinoplasty Can Improve:

- Deviated septum correction (septoplasty) to improve airflow through both nostrils.
- Nasal valve reinforcement to prevent collapse when breathing in deeply.
- Turbinate reduction to create more space in the airway.
- Post-traumatic nasal deformity repair to restore breathing after injury.

What Rhinoplasty Won't Fix:

- Allergies or chronic inflammation (requires medical treatment).
- Nasal polyps or sinus issues (may need separate sinus surgery).
- Mouth breathing due to habit or anatomical issues outside the nose.

Many patients don't realize how much their nasal anatomy affects their quality of life until it's corrected. And the best part? Once function is restored, the benefits last a lifetime.

The Balance of Form and Function

A truly successful rhinoplasty isn't just about creating a nose that looks good, it's about creating one that functions beautifully, too. The best aesthetic result is one that looks effortless and natural, while allowing the patient to breathe freely, sleep better, and feel more energized.

This is why every rhinoplasty should begin with a thorough evaluation of both external structure and internal airway function. A nose that photographs well but doesn't breathe well is a flawed outcome.

In the end, what good is a beautiful nose if you can't breathe through it?

CHAPTER 12
WHAT IS THE BEST AGE FOR RHINOPLASTY?

When Is the Right Time for a Rhinoplasty?
One of the most common questions I hear from patients—and often from their parents—is, "What is the right age for a nose job?"

The short answer is that it depends.

After performing thousands of rhinoplasties, I can confidently say there is no single perfect age, only the right time for each individual. Some patients seek refinement in their teenage years, others wait until their late twenties or thirties, and some finally decide in their fifties or sixties. Your nose is with you for life, and the best time to undergo rhinoplasty is when you are truly ready—physically, emotionally, and mentally.

While age alone does not dictate readiness, different stages of life bring unique considerations. Let's explore the most common age groups for rhinoplasty and what each one entails.

· · ·

Teenage Rhinoplasty: The Most Common Age Group
For many who eventually pursue rhinoplasty, the first thoughts of altering their nose arise around the ages of ten or eleven. At this stage, children become more aware of their features and how they compare to their peers. Some feel self-conscious about a dorsal hump, a wide tip, or asymmetry, though their nose is still in development. By the mid-teen years, the decision becomes more serious.

For girls, rhinoplasty is generally safe by the age of fifteen, once facial growth is complete. Boys tend to grow slightly longer, making sixteen or later a more appropriate age.

Many teenage patients want surgery before their senior year of high school. They see it as a fresh start—an opportunity to begin college with a nose that feels right for them, without the baggage of childhood teasing or self-consciousness. They hope to avoid awkward questions or unsolicited comments from classmates and instead enter a new phase of life with quiet confidence.

When performed for the right reasons, rhinoplasty can be truly transformative for young patients. But it is a decision that demands careful thought. Before I operate on a teenager, I ensure they are emotionally mature enough to make the decision for themselves, that they fully understand the healing process and what to expect, and, most importantly, that they are choosing surgery for themselves, not because of peer pressure or family influence.

· · ·

A Conversation with Parents

Parents often hesitate when their child expresses a desire for rhinoplasty. Some worry that it's an unnecessary cosmetic procedure. Others feel protective, insisting their child is beautiful as they are. They may say, "Why change something natural?" or "You're too young to make such a big decision."

These concerns are valid, but what parents sometimes fail to recognize is the deep emotional impact a nose can have on a young person's confidence. This is not about vanity. It's about how a teenager feels when they step into a room, when they take a photo, when they catch their reflection unexpectedly. Some teenagers simply dislike their nose. Others suffer because of it. The distinction is crucial. We will explore this more in Chapter 29.

The Girl Who Couldn't Wait

I generally do not operate on patients younger than fifteen. But every so often, there are exceptions.

A fourteen-year-old girl sat across from me in my office, her shoulders drawn in, eyes fixed on her lap. She barely spoke. It was her mother who explained why they were there.

"She has been begging us for this for years," she said. "She gets bullied every day at school. The kids call her 'witch nose.' She doesn't want to go to school anymore."

I turned to the girl. "Is that true?" She nodded without looking up. "I just don't want to look like this anymore."

When I examined her, I saw that her facial growth was complete. Medically, she was ready. Emotionally, she needed this.

Operating on young patients is a decision I take seriously, and I never recommend surgery unless I believe it is truly in the patient's best interest. In her case, the psychological burden of waiting outweighed the risks of early surgery. After a long discussion with her and her parents about expectations, recovery, and healing, we scheduled her procedure.

A few months later, she walked into my office for a follow-up, and I hardly recognized her. She carried herself differently—shoulders back, head high, an unmistakable lightness in her expression.

"I'm happy," she said simply. For her, the timing was right.

Young Adulthood: The "I Always Wanted to Do This" Group
By their twenties, many patients have been considering rhinoplasty for years but have waited until they were fully grown or financially independent to pursue it. Some say they always knew they wanted to refine their nose but felt more confident making the decision as an adult. Others had parents who were hesitant to approve surgery as teenagers and now, for the first time, can make the choice on their own.

At this stage in life, patients typically have a stable sense of self, a clear understanding of their features, and the means to invest in a procedure they have long considered. After surgery, many express a feeling of alignment between their inner and outer selves. They no longer fixate on their nose in photos or avoid certain angles in mirrors. Instead, they feel at ease, as if their nose has always belonged to them.

Rhinoplasty Later in Life: The "I Wish I Had Done This Sooner" Group

There are those who wait decades before finally deciding to undergo rhinoplasty. Some have wanted it since they were young but put it off due to life circumstances—career, family, or simply the fear of change. Others seek surgery not because they always disliked their nose, but because it has changed with age.

Over time, nasal cartilage weakens, the tip may begin to droop, and the skin may thin, revealing more of the underlying structure. For these patients, rhinoplasty is not about erasing the past but restoring balance and harmony to their features. Many choose to combine their procedure with a facelift, ensuring that their nose and face age in harmony.

After surgery, the most common sentiment I hear from this group is regret—not over having the procedure, but over waiting so long to do it. "I finally put myself first," they say. "I look like me, just refreshed."

Does the Nose Change with Age?

Yes, though not in the way many people assume. The bones remain the same, but the soft tissues shift over time.

The tip may begin to droop due to weakened cartilage. The nose may appear longer as the ligaments loosen. In some cases, the skin becomes thinner, making the underlying structures more pronounced.

CHAPTER 13

WHY REVISION RHINOPLASTY IS MORE COMPLEX

When patients come in for a consultation about revision rhinoplasty, they are often surprised—sometimes even shocked—by what they hear.

"Wait, why does a revision take longer?"
"Why does it cost more?"
"Why is the healing harder than the first time?"

These are fair questions. Most people assume that a revision is just another attempt at their original surgery, a quick fix to correct what didn't turn out right the first time. But nothing could be further from the truth. Revision rhinoplasty is not simply a do-over, it's a meticulous reconstruction that requires careful planning, patience, and, above all, the right mindset.

I've seen this realization dawn on many patients, but one story, in particular, stands out.

• • •

Sarah's Story: A Second Chance at the Nose She Always Wanted

Sarah came into my office at twenty-six, a decade after her first rhinoplasty. She had undergone surgery at sixteen—an age when she had little say in the process. Her mother had arranged the procedure with a local plastic surgeon, the same one who had performed her mother's facelift a few years before.

"I thought I was getting the nose of my dreams," she told me, frustration lacing her voice. *"But it just… never felt right."*

At first glance, Sarah's nose wasn't an obvious case for revision. It wasn't severely misshapen or drastically overdone. But something was off. The tip lacked definition, the bridge had been over-reduced, and subtle irregularities gave her profile a slightly collapsed look. More than anything, she felt that her nose didn't belong to her.

"I just want a second chance," she said. *"I want to get it right this time."*

As we talked, it became clear that she believed revision rhinoplasty would be just like her first surgery—same process, same expectations, same recovery. The only difference, in her mind, was that this time, she had chosen a better surgeon.

I had to pause.

· · ·

"*Sarah,*" I said gently, "*this is not the same as your first surgery. A revision isn't just another shot at a primary rhinoplasty—it's an entirely different surgery, with different rules.*"

She frowned. "*But…it's still just reshaping the nose, right?*"

I could see she needed time to absorb this. So we didn't just talk once—we had multiple conversations, over several sessions, until she fully understood what she was signing up for.

The Hidden Complexities of Revision Rhinoplasty
What Sarah didn't realize—and what many revision patients don't—is that once a nose has been operated on, it is never the same again.

<u>The Anatomy Is No Longer "Normal"</u>
In primary rhinoplasty, I work with untouched tissue, natural cartilage, and skin that has never been lifted or repositioned. It's like sculpting a statue from a fresh block of marble.

But in a revision case, the original structure has already been altered. Cartilage may have been removed, leaving the nose structurally weak. Scar tissue may have formed, fusing layers together in unpredictable ways. The skin may have lost elasticity, making it less forgiving. The surgical approach in these cases isn't just about reshaping, it's about rebuilding.

• • •

The Surgery Itself Takes Longer

Sarah was stunned when I told her that her revision surgery would take nearly twice as long as a primary rhinoplasty.

"Why?" she asked. *"Isn't it just a matter of fixing what was done before?"*

Not quite. Revision surgery demands far more meticulous work than a first-time rhinoplasty. Every step takes longer.

Dissecting through scar tissue requires extreme precision because, instead of smooth, natural planes, I must navigate areas that have unpredictably healed together. If too much cartilage was removed in the first surgery, I may need to harvest cartilage from the ear or even the rib to restore structure. In many cases, I don't fully know what was done before until I'm inside the nose, which means every revision surgery requires adaptability—no two are ever the same.

Sarah had no idea how much was involved. But once she understood, she realized this wasn't a minor correction, it was a full reconstruction.

Healing Takes Longer—And It's Different This Time

When Sarah had her first rhinoplasty at sixteen, her recovery was relatively smooth. Swelling went down in a few months, and by the one-year mark, she had moved on. She assumed it would be the same this time.

· · ·

It wouldn't be.

Revision surgery involves working with scarred tissue and altered anatomy, which means swelling lasts longer. Fluid drainage isn't as efficient as in a first-time rhinoplasty, so the nose holds onto swelling for an extended period. The nasal skin, already stretched and manipulated from the first surgery, doesn't behave the same way. Perhaps most frustratingly, the healing process can feel unpredictable—some days, the nose looks great, and then, suddenly, swelling flares up for no apparent reason.

"Sarah, you need to be prepared for this," I told her. *"There will be moments when you question whether you made the right decision. And that's completely normal. The key is to trust the process."*

She nodded, taking it in. This time, she wasn't a teenager being led into surgery—she was making an informed decision for herself.

Sarah's Surgery—and Why She Succeeded

The day of Sarah's surgery, all the complexities I had warned her about were there.

We encountered significant scar tissue along the bridge that had to be carefully released. The tip lacked proper support, requiring cartilage grafting to restore structure. The skin was less elastic than I would have liked, so we had to be even more meticulous in redraping it.

But we navigated each challenge, step by step. When Sarah finally saw her new nose, she was overwhelmed.

"It's me," she said, her eyes filling with tears. *"For the first time, it actually feels like my nose."*

Of course, the journey wasn't over. There was still swelling to manage, follow-ups to attend, patience to maintain. But because she had gone into surgery with the right mindset, she wasn't discouraged by the slow healing. She expected it. She understood it. And she trusted the process. That made all the difference.

Final Thoughts: The Power of Knowledge
Sarah's story is a perfect example of why education is critical in revision rhinoplasty. If she had gone into surgery thinking it would be quick and easy, she would have struggled through recovery, second-guessed every bump, and panicked over every fluctuation.

That anxiety could have negatively impacted her results—because stress affects healing, and impatience can lead to poor post-operative decisions. But because she knew what to expect, she succeeded.

· · ·

That's why I always emphasize knowledge before surgery. Revision rhinoplasty is not for everyone. It's more complex and requires more patience. It is more expensive. But when done right, in the right hands, it can be life-changing.

PART 2: THE ART AND SCIENCE OF RHINOPLASTY

CHAPTER 14
THE TRUTH ABOUT NONSURGICAL RHINOPLASTY: ILLUSION, RISKS, AND THE LONG-TERM IMPACT

Over the past decade, more and more patients have turned to nonsurgical rhinoplasty as a quick fix for nasal refinement. I get it—the idea of enhancing your nose without surgery is appealing. The procedure is marketed as fast, painless, and reversible, a way to "try out" a new nose without the commitment of surgery. But what many patients don't realize is that, like everything in aesthetics, nonsurgical rhinoplasty has its place and its limitations.

It's a useful tool, but it's not magic. And in the wrong hands, it can cause more harm than good.

Unlike surgical rhinoplasty, which physically reshapes the nose, nonsurgical rhinoplasty works by masking irregularities rather than modifying underlying structure. It's an illusion—an effective one in the right cases, but still an illusion. The challenge is many patients don't fully understand what this means. They assume that if filler can make the nose look straighter, smaller, or more refined, it must work the same way as surgery. But it doesn't. And before considering it, it's important to understand what it can—and can't—do.

How Nonsurgical Rhinoplasty Works

The procedure relies on injectable fillers, most commonly hyaluronic acid, to reshape the nose by adding volume to specific areas. A carefully placed injection at the bridge can smooth out a small hump, making the nose appear straighter. A subtle amount of filler at the tip can give the illusion of more projection. By manipulating how light reflects off the nose, the overall structure can appear more sculpted and balanced.

This effect is purely visual. Fillers do not change nasal structure. They do not reduce size, correct deviations, or improve function. Instead, they work by shifting proportions, creating an optical trick that makes the nose appear more refined.

The entire procedure takes just a few minutes, with results visible almost immediately. In some cases, botulinum toxin can be used alongside filler to enhance results. For example, relaxing the depressor septi muscle—which pulls the nasal tip downward when smiling or speaking—can create a slight lifting effect. It's a subtle improvement, but temporary, lasting only a few months before the muscle regains function.

While these techniques can offer impressive refinements in the right patient, the growing popularity of nonsurgical rhinoplasty has led to an explosion of treatments that push beyond what fillers were ever meant to do.

. . .

One trend I strongly discourage is thread lifts for nasal refinement. I have removed countless threads from patients' noses during rhinoplasty, and the amount of scarring and fibrosis they leave behind is significant. Despite being marketed as a minimally invasive way to refine the nose, they create more problems than they solve—not just in the nose, but anywhere in the face.

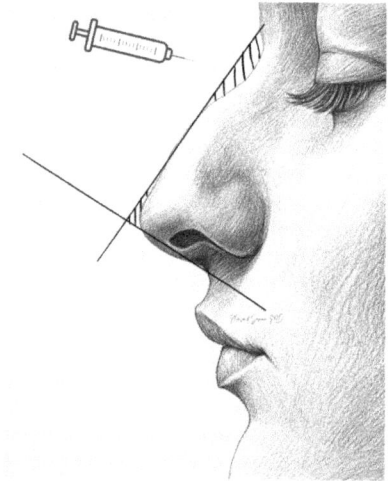

Strategic placement of dermal fillers can create a straighter bridge and improve tip projection and position.

The Limitations of Nonsurgical Rhinoplasty

For all the optical refinements filler can provide, it has clear limitations.

Many patients believe it can make their nose smaller, but it can't. Fillers add volume. They cannot reduce size, only create the appearance of refinement. They can smooth out a hump but won't make a nose less prominent. They can camouflage minor asymmetries but won't straighten a truly crooked nose.

Perhaps most importantly, nonsurgical rhinoplasty does nothing to improve breathing. Unlike surgical rhinoplasty, which can correct a deviated septum or reinforce nasal valves to prevent collapse, filler has no impact on airflow.

Then there's the issue of permanence. While fillers are often marketed as "temporary," some patients undergo repeated treatments for years, unknowingly accumulating long-term changes to their nasal structure. Over time, filler can migrate, stretch tissues, and make future surgery more complicated.

One of the biggest misconceptions I hear is that filler can "shrink" a nose. It can't. What it does exceptionally well, however, is trick the eye. By strategically placing filler, we can manipulate shadows and highlights to create a more balanced appearance. But at the end of the day, it's an illusion. Patients expecting a nonsurgical nose job to actually reduce their nose size will always be disappointed.

When a Quick Fix Becomes a Long-Term Problem: Sheena's Story

Sheena had never liked her nose. Even as a child, she would tilt her head at certain angles in the mirror, trying to imagine what it would look like if it were just a little different. But surgery? That had always felt too extreme. The idea of anesthesia, downtime, and permanent change made her uneasy.

. . .

Then she discovered nonsurgical rhinoplasty.

"It was so easy," she told me. "I'd get a little touch-up, and I'd walk out looking better instantly."

For nearly ten years, she followed this routine—a quick appointment, a few injections, an immediate confidence boost. It became second nature. Until, one day, it wasn't.

At first, it was just slight tenderness. Then, a darkening of the skin. By the next day, it hurt—badly. That's when the panic set in.

By the time she came to me, she was at serious risk of losing skin on her nose. A blood vessel had been inadvertently occluded—meaning the filler had blocked circulation to her skin. Worse still, her injector had used a non-dissolvable filler, so there was no way to quickly reverse the damage.

Had she received a dissolvable filler, I could have injected an enzyme called hyaluronidase, which restores blood flow within minutes. But in her case, we were forced to rely on emergency treatments—nitroglycerin paste, warm compresses, and circulation-boosting interventions.

We were able to salvage the skin, but the damage had already been done. The long-term effects of vascular compromise meant that her options for future surgery were now limited. Instead of a full structural rhinoplasty, we had to take a preservation approach, working around the areas of previous damage.

Sheena was lucky. Not everyone is.

The Psychological Trap of Nonsurgical Rhinoplasty
One of the reasons nonsurgical rhinoplasty has exploded in popularity is that it allows patients to "try out" a new nose with low commitment. But what many don't realize is that constantly tweaking their nose with filler can distort their perception of what looks natural.

I've seen patients who start with a minor tweak but, over time, become hyper-focused on their nose, always seeking just a little more. The problem is that repeated filler injections can subtly distort facial balance. A small enhancement today might look great, but after years of layering filler on top of filler, the nose can start looking unnatural—especially when the filler moves or settles in unexpected ways.

This is why I always discuss long-term goals with patients, not just the immediate results.

Final Thoughts: Is Nonsurgical Rhinoplasty Right for You?
For the right patient, nonsurgical rhinoplasty can be a powerful tool. It's best suited for those looking for subtle refinements, temporary enhancements for an event, or minor touch-ups after surgery.

• • •

It's not a substitute for traditional rhinoplasty. It cannot make the nose smaller, improve function, or provide a long-term solution for patients who want permanent refinement.

More importantly, it carries risks. Unlike filler in the lips or cheeks, where misplaced injections are rarely serious, filler in the nose is high-risk. The blood supply to the nose is fragile, and a poorly placed injection can block circulation, leading to skin death or even blindness.

That's why who performs the procedure matters. Many injectors offering nonsurgical rhinoplasty are not nasal specialists. Some have taken only a weekend course on fillers before offering the treatment in their practice. But understanding nasal anatomy is critical.

In the right hands, nonsurgical rhinoplasty can be a safe, effective enhancement. In the wrong hands, it can complicate the future of your nose forever.

CHAPTER 15
THE NOSE IN FACIAL HARMONY: THE ART OF BALANCE

A well-proportioned nose is never just about the nose itself. It exists within the context of the entire face, and its beauty lies in how seamlessly it blends with the surrounding features. Patients often come to me with a singular focus—a dorsal hump, a drooping tip, a width that feels too broad. But the truth is, achieving a natural and elegant result requires stepping back and considering the face as a whole.

This is why my consultations extend far beyond just the nose. I take time to analyze the proportions, contours, and relationships between facial features, because a nose that is technically refined but out of sync with the rest of the face does not create true beauty.

Facial Proportions: A Delicate Balance

Many subtle yet powerful factors influence how a nose appears within a face. Understanding these nuances is essential to achieving harmony rather than simply chasing a mathematically "straight" or "small" nose.

Facial asymmetry is a key consideration. Nearly every face has some degree of imbalance, and sometimes, the nose appears off-center not because it is actually crooked, but because the underlying facial bones are asymmetric. A well-planned rhinoplasty must work with these natural variations rather than forcing an artificial straightness that may not suit the face.

Chin projection also plays a major role. A small or recessed chin can create the illusion of a nose that looks too large. In many cases, a patient may believe their nose needs to be dramatically reduced, when in reality, a subtle chin enhancement could bring the entire face into better proportion.

The contour of the forehead affects how the nasal bridge is perceived. A high or prominent forehead can make a nose look more delicate, while a flatter forehead can create a sharper transition into the nasal bridge, altering the profile's overall balance.

Even the relationship between the nose and the mouth matters. A long upper lip can appear even longer if the nasal tip is lifted too much, changing the proportions of the lower face. If a patient already has minimal tooth show at rest, lifting the nasal tip too aggressively could result in a less youthful, even stern, appearance.

· · ·

A beautiful nose is never just about the nose, it's about how it fits within the entire face.

These are just a few of the many factors that must be assessed during a proper rhinoplasty evaluation. Every face has unique angles, proportions, and asymmetries, and each surgical plan must be meticulously tailored to maintain balance and harmony.

Full Facial Analysis

I often see a moment of hesitation in my patients' eyes when I begin discussing their chin, forehead, or lip position during a rhinoplasty consultation. Their expression sometimes carries an unspoken question: *Why are we talking about this? I just want to fix my nose.* But as we delve deeper, it becomes clear—the goal is not just to refine the nose, but to create harmony across the entire face.

This is why I take the time to perform a comprehensive facial analysis before making any recommendations. True aesthetic enhancement is not about changing one feature in isolation, it's about ensuring that every adjustment respects the natural flow and balance of the face.

The Goal: Refinement, Not Just Reduction

The best rhinoplasties do not draw attention. They do not make people say, "Nice nose job." Instead, they elicit a sense of balance and effortless beauty, where no single feature overpowers another. A well-executed rhinoplasty does not stand alone, it integrates seamlessly into the face, enhancing the patient's natural character rather than altering it.

· · ·

This is why rhinoplasty is not just a surgical procedure, but a discipline of proportion, symmetry, and artistry. It is not simply about reducing a hump or refining a tip, it's about creating a nose that belongs to the face, a nose that enhances rather than distracts. This can only be achieved when we take into account every angle, every contour, and every subtle relationship that defines the individual beauty of each patient.

CHAPTER 16
HOW TO PREPARE FOR YOUR RHINOPLASTY CONSULTATION

This chapter is designed to equip you with the knowledge and confidence to navigate your rhinoplasty consultation with ease. The goal is not just to find a qualified surgeon but to find the right surgeon for you —one who understands your vision, communicates openly, and has the experience to achieve a result that complements your natural features. A well-prepared consultation ensures you walk away informed, assured, and clear on whether this is the right step for you.

It's wise to meet with at least two, ideally three, surgeons before making a final decision. Each consultation offers a different perspective, giving you a broader understanding of what's possible and allowing you to assess surgical styles, bedside manner, and overall approach. The right choice is about more than credentials, it's about trust and alignment in aesthetic goals.

———

Researching Your Surgeon

Before setting foot in a consultation room, take the time to research your potential surgeons. Verify that they are board-certified in facial plastic surgery or plastic surgery and have extensive experience with rhinoplasty. Check their state medical license and professional society memberships, such as the American Academy of Facial Plastic and Reconstructive Surgery. Beyond credentials, carefully study their before-and-after photos—do the results look natural? Do they align with your aesthetic preferences? The goal is to find a surgeon whose work reflects precision, artistry, and balance.

Learning from Other Patients

Patient testimonials can offer valuable insight into a surgeon's approach, skill, and the overall experience they provide. While online reviews are helpful, speaking directly to previous patients—if possible—can give a deeper understanding of the process, from consultation to recovery. Ask about their satisfaction with their results, how the office handled their concerns, and whether they felt supported throughout the journey.

Preparing for a Revision Rhinoplasty Consultation

If you are considering a revision rhinoplasty, preparation is key. Bring before and after photos from your first surgery to help the surgeon understand your concerns. If possible, obtain operative notes from your previous procedure—these records can provide crucial information on what was done initially and guide the revision approach.

Considering Previous Nonsurgical Rhinoplasty (Filler)

If you have had a nonsurgical rhinoplasty using filler, it's best to dissolve it before your consultation so the surgeon can assess your natural nasal structure. If dissolving isn't feasible before your appointment, bring a photo of your nose before filler to give the surgeon a more accurate reference point.

Using Inspiration Photos Wisely

Bringing inspiration photos can be helpful, but they should serve as a general guide rather than an exact blueprint. Keep in mind that no two faces are the same, and a nose that looks great on someone else may not be the best fit for your facial harmony. A skilled surgeon will consider your unique features and work toward a result that enhances your natural beauty rather than replicating someone else's.

Evaluating Your Surgeon During the Consultation

Your consultation is an opportunity to assess not only the surgeon's technical expertise but also their philosophy and communication style. Ask yourself:

- Do they listen attentively and address my concerns?
- Do they explain their approach clearly and honestly?
- Do I feel comfortable discussing my goals with them?
- Does their past work reflect the level of artistry I'm seeking?

The best surgeons combine skill with an ability to collaborate and guide their patients toward the best possible outcomes.

. . .

Asking the Right Questions

A well-prepared patient asks direct and thoughtful questions. Consider asking:

- How many rhinoplasties do you perform each year?
- What percentage of your practice is focused on rhinoplasty?
- What is your preferred surgical approach—preservation, structural, ultrasonic, or a combination?
- Can you show me before-and-after photos of patients with similar features to mine?
- How do you handle revisions if I'm not satisfied with the result?
- What are the specific challenges or limitations of my nose?
- What should I expect in terms of healing time and final results?
- Do you use internal packing or splints?
- What type of anesthesia do you use, and who administers it?
- How do you determine whether my desired result will suit my facial structure?

Understanding Costs and Policies

Surgical expertise comes at a cost, and it's important to understand the financial aspect upfront. Ask for a detailed breakdown of expenses, including the surgical fee, facility fee, anesthesia, and post-operative care. Inquire about payment options and financing plans, and clarify the revision policy—some surgeons offer minor adjustments at a reduced rate, while others charge full price for any revisions.

• • •

Planning for Recovery

Recovery is an important part of the process and understanding what to expect can help you prepare accordingly. Ask about:

- Expected swelling, bruising, and healing milestones
- Activity restrictions (exercise, sun exposure, wearing glasses)
- Post-operative care instructions (nasal taping, lymphatic massage, medications)

Knowing what to expect post-surgery will help set realistic expectations and ease the recovery journey.

Exploring Technology & Imaging Tools

Some surgeons offer digital morphing or 3D imaging to simulate potential results. While these tools can be useful, remember that they are approximations, not guarantees. Ask how your surgeon uses these tools in planning and whether they find them reliable for setting expectations.

Clarifying Who Will Perform the Surgery

Ensure that the surgeon you are consulting with is the one who will be performing your procedure, rather than a fellow or resident. Ask about the role of assistants or surgical team members and what aspects of the procedure they may be involved in.

Assessing the Surgical Facility

The setting of your surgery matters. Ask if the facility is accredited (e.g., AAAASF, JCAHO) and about their infection control and emergency protocols. A well-run surgical center with high safety standards is just as critical as the surgeon's expertise.

Managing Expectations and Emotional Readiness

Rhinoplasty is not just a physical change, it's a process that requires patience and mental readiness. Expect fluctuations in your emotions, especially in the early recovery phase when swelling is still present. The best results take time, and it's important to trust the process.

Timing Your Procedure

Many top surgeons book out months in advance, so plan accordingly. Consider factors like work and social obligations when choosing your surgery date. Some patients prefer winter recovery when social events are fewer, while others schedule around life milestones.

Reflecting on Your Decision

After completing your consultations, take time to reflect. Ask yourself:

- Which surgeon made me feel the most confident in their skills?
- Who took the time to understand my goals and concerns?
- Do I trust this surgeon's aesthetic judgment and surgical ability?

Your choice should be based on a balance of expertise, artistic vision, and trust. Take your time, weigh your options, and make the decision that feels right for you.

• • •

Final Thoughts

The consultation is your chance to gather knowledge, explore possibilities, and make an informed decision about your rhinoplasty journey. The best outcomes come from a collaboration between patient and surgeon, built on trust, transparency, and shared vision. By preparing well and asking the right questions, you take control of your journey and set the stage for a successful, beautifully natural result.

CHAPTER 17
COMPUTER SIMULATIONS AND 3D MODELS

What if you could see your new nose before surgery? With today's digital simulations and 3D modeling, this is possible. But how accurate are these previews? More importantly—should you trust them?

Technology has transformed the way we approach rhinoplasty. These digital tools allow patients to visualize potential changes, helping bridge the gap between expectation and reality. They provide a blueprint, a way to align the surgeon's vision with the patient's desires.

As with any tool, there are limitations. A simulation is not a promise, and it certainly isn't a crystal ball. The human body is not a static, digital object—it is dynamic, living tissue that heals and settles in ways that no software can fully predict. This is why I always encourage patients to approach simulations as a guide, not as an absolute guarantee of what their final nose will look like.

. . .

The Power—and Limits—of Digital Imaging

There is something inherently exciting about seeing a preview of what your new nose could look like. I see it all the time—when a patient sees their simulated result, their eyes light up with possibility. For some, it's the first time they've ever envisioned themselves without the feature that has long bothered them.

However, I always remind patients: *Take this with a grain of salt.* The purpose of a digital simulation is to provide aesthetic direction, not an exact roadmap. It helps us refine proportions, angles, and overall balance, but it cannot account for the subtle, organic qualities of real human anatomy. Skin thickness, cartilage memory, healing patterns, and even the way light interacts with the skin all contribute to the final result in ways that a screen simply cannot replicate.

Some simulation software produces results that are too perfect, with artificially smoothed contours and poreless skin. These images may look appealing, but they create unrealistic expectations. A real nose will always have natural variations, texture, and the subtle asymmetries that define human beauty.

How Artificial Intelligence Enhances My Approach

While digital imaging is valuable, I take it a step further by incorporating AI-driven facial analysis into my consultations.

Artificial intelligence allows me to objectively assess nasal proportions, symmetry, and facial balance in a way that the human eye alone may not always capture. This scientific framework provides a starting point, offering a structural breakdown of what might enhance harmony.

But AI doesn't just analyze symmetry, it evaluates proportion, balance, and even how different angles affect perception. Yet, AI alone isn't enough. It can suggest the mathematically 'ideal' nose, but beauty isn't just about ratios, it's about character, personality, and the subtleties that make a face uniquely beautiful. That's why I use AI as a tool, not a decision-maker.

Once we have this objective analysis, I sit with the patient and add the human element—our shared aesthetic vision. Some patients want a nose that reflects idealized proportions, while others want to preserve certain ethnic or characteristic features. AI gives us the objective foundation, but together, we craft the artistic execution.

Why I Ask Patients to Bring Their Own Digital Edits
In today's world, patients are more visually engaged with their desired aesthetic than ever before. Many experiment with filters, FaceTune, or Photoshop, adjusting their own images to see how a refined nose might change their appearance.

I encourage patients to bring these edited images to their consultation—not because we will replicate them exactly, but because they provide valuable insight into their personal aesthetic preferences. By analyzing what a patient has altered, I can better understand the level of refinement they're seeking, whether they prefer a soft, natural look or a more sculpted, defined aesthetic. These images also reveal their perception of facial balance. Sometimes, patients are drawn to exaggerated edits that wouldn't translate naturally in real life, which leads to an important discussion about realistic and achievable results.

Rather than setting unrealistic expectations, these images serve as a starting point for conversation, helping me align their vision with what is surgically possible while ensuring their results enhance their natural beauty.

Why I also Ask for Photos of Noses They *Dislike*

Equally important as knowing what a patient wants is knowing what they don't want. I always ask my patients to bring examples of rhinoplasty results they dislike. This might seem unusual at first, but it often tells me more than the images they admire.

Understanding what a patient finds unattractive is just as important as knowing what they desire. It helps me recognize their aesthetic boundaries—what feels like "too much" or "not enough" to them. Some may worry about an over-reduced nose, an excessively rotated tip, or losing the natural character of their nose. Others have a specific idea of what looks "unnatural," a perception that varies greatly from person to person.

By discussing both positive and negative visual references, we create a more precise and meaningful dialogue. This ensures that the patient and I are fully aligned before surgery, minimizing the risk of miscommunication and allowing for results that feel both intentional and authentic to them.

Digital Previews Are a Guide, Not a Guarantee
I tell my patients this often: *Your final nose will be real, not digital.* It will move, breathe, and shift subtly as it heals. It will have natural variations in texture, light reflection, and symmetry.

Computer simulations and 3D models are incredibly valuable tools, but they should be viewed as aesthetic blueprints, not contracts. They provide a visual roadmap, but just like any journey, there are natural variables along the way. By combining technology, AI analysis, and human artistry, we can refine a plan that aligns with a patient's expectations while remaining grounded in what is actually achievable.

At the end of the day, your final nose won't be a digital rendering on a screen, it will be a living, breathing part of you. No simulation, no matter how advanced, can fully predict the way a nose will integrate with your features or the confidence that comes from a result that feels authentically yours.

Surgery is only one half of the journey. The other half lies in healing, a process that unfolds uniquely in every individual. No technology can account for the nuances of tissue response, swelling resolution, or how your body ultimately settles into its new shape. The best predictor of your outcome isn't a computer-generated image, it's your surgeon's experience. Their skill, their understanding of anatomy, and their track record with patients who share similar features to yours are what truly guide realistic expectations.

CHAPTER 18
OPEN VS. CLOSED RHINOPLASTY – THE DIFFERENCES, PROS, AND CONS

Open vs. Closed Rhinoplasty: Choosing the Right Approach

One of the most debated topics in rhinoplasty is whether open or closed rhinoplasty is the better approach. Patients often ask, "Which one is better?" or assume that closed rhinoplasty is superior simply because it leaves no external scar. Even among surgeons, opinions vary widely, often shaped by their training rather than objective differences between the techniques.

The truth is, both methods are far more similar than most people think. While many believe that open rhinoplasty offers better visualization or that closed rhinoplasty is always less invasive, these are misconceptions rather than absolute truths. As a surgeon experienced in both techniques, I choose my approach based on the patient's unique anatomy, surgical goals, and long-term outcome, not a rigid preference for one method over the other.

. . .

Understanding these two approaches is key to setting realistic expectations and ensuring the best surgical plan for each individual patient.

What is Open Rhinoplasty?

Open rhinoplasty involves a small incision across the columella—the strip of skin between the nostrils. This allows the nasal skin to be lifted, providing direct access to the bone and cartilage. The primary advantage of this approach is unobstructed visibility, which can be particularly useful for complex cases requiring significant structural work.

For patients with thick skin, an open approach allows for internal thinning before redraping, which can improve definition in the final result. It's also the preferred technique when extensive modifications are needed, such as major tip refinement, grafting, severe asymmetry correction, or nasal valve repair to improve breathing.

Revision rhinoplasty is another scenario where I always opt for an open approach. When working through scar tissue from previous surgeries, having full access to the underlying structures allows for more precise reconstruction and stabilization.

The trade-off? A small external incision on the columella. In most cases, this heals exceptionally well and becomes nearly imperceptible over time. If needed, laser treatments or scar refinement techniques can further minimize visibility. The other consideration is initial swelling, particularly in the nasal tip, which may take a little longer to subside compared to closed rhinoplasty. However, in the long run, the final healing process and results are the same for both techniques.

What is Closed (Endonasal) Rhinoplasty?

Closed rhinoplasty, also called endonasal rhinoplasty, involves making all incisions inside the nostrils, leaving no external scar. Contrary to popular belief—even among some surgeons—this approach does not inherently mean poorer visibility or less precision. With modern instrumentation and technique, a well-executed closed rhinoplasty can provide just as much control and refinement as an open approach in many cases.

For patients seeking hump reduction, minor tip refinement, or adjustments to the nasal bridge, closed rhinoplasty can be a great option. Keeping the skin partially attached preserves blood supply, which may help minimize initial swelling. Patients with thin skin often benefit from a closed approach as well, as it allows the skin to redrape more naturally over the refined structure.

However, closed rhinoplasty does have limitations. Certain procedures—such as extensive tip reshaping, major grafting, or correction of complex asymmetries—can be more challenging without full exposure. In patients with thick skin, I often prefer an open approach to allow for more internal sculpting.

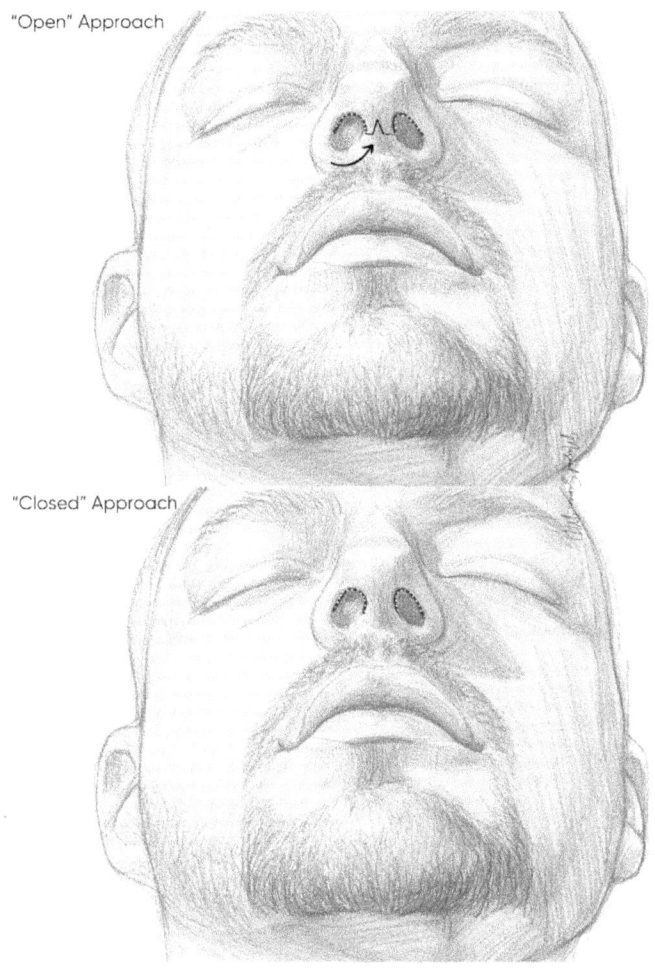

Schematic of incision placement for open rhinoplasty (top) and closed rhinoplasty (bottom)

Are Open and Closed Techniques Really That Different?

Many surgeons trained exclusively in open rhinoplasty believe it provides better visualization and control. While this may be true for some cases, a properly executed closed rhinoplasty can achieve the same level of precision in the right hands.

Similarly, many patients assume that closed rhinoplasty is always less invasive and leads to a faster recovery. This isn't entirely accurate. The invasiveness of a rhinoplasty depends more on what's being done inside the nose rather than whether the incisions are internal or external.

For example, a closed rhinoplasty that requires significant restructuring can be just as invasive as an open approach. And while tip swelling may linger slightly longer after open rhinoplasty, the overall healing timeline for both techniques is more similar than most patients expect.

How I Decide Which Approach to Use

Because I perform both open and closed rhinoplasty, I select the technique based on what will yield the best long-term result for the patient. My decision is guided by several factors:

- The Patient's Anatomy – In patients with thick skin, an open approach allows for internal thinning, which can enhance definition.
- The Complexity of the Surgery – If extensive sculpting of the nasal tip, major grafting, or significant sidewall modifications are needed, open rhinoplasty may be the better choice.

- Whether it's a Revision Case – I always use an open approach for revisions, as it allows for precise removal of scar tissue and structural reinforcement.
- The Patient's Goals – For those seeking subtle refinements with minimal disruption, closed rhinoplasty may be ideal.
- Ultimately, the technique should serve the patient's needs, not the surgeon's preference.

Common Myths About Open vs. Closed Rhinoplasty

A few misconceptions about these approaches continue to persist:

"Closed rhinoplasty is always less invasive."
Not necessarily. A closed rhinoplasty can be just as invasive if major structural changes are needed.
"Open rhinoplasty always leads to a longer recovery."
While tip swelling may take slightly longer to subside, the final healing process is the same for both techniques.
"Closed rhinoplasty is always better because there's no scar."
The small columellar incision in open rhinoplasty is usually imperceptible, and the improved access may outweigh the concern in more complex cases.

Final Thoughts: The Right Approach for the Right Patient

There is no universal "best" technique in rhinoplasty. Both open and closed approaches have their place in modern nasal surgery. What truly matters is selecting the method that will deliver the most refined, natural, and lasting result for each patient.

For me, long-term results always take priority over surgical preference. My decision is based on:

- The patient's anatomy

- The complexity of the procedure
- The balance between control and healing

At the end of the day, the technique is just a tool. What truly determines success isn't whether a rhinoplasty is open or closed—it's whether it is performed with expertise, precision, and a deep understanding of both form and function.

CHAPTER 19
PRESERVATION RHINOPLASTY VS. STRUCTURAL RHINOPLASTY: AN OVERVIEW

Rhinoplasty is not a one-size-fits-all procedure. Every nose is unique, and over time, surgical techniques have evolved to offer different approaches depending on a patient's anatomy, goals, and functional needs.

For much of the 20th century, rhinoplasty primarily followed a structural approach. If a patient had a hump, it was shaved down; if refinement was needed, cartilage was removed, repositioned, or reinforced with grafts. This method became widely used because of its predictability and ability to create stable, long-term results.

At the same time, other surgeons maintained a different philosophy—one that sought to preserve as much of the natural nasal framework as possible while still achieving refinement. Rather than removing a hump, for example, preservation rhinoplasty lowers the bridge from beneath, maintaining the continuity of the nasal dorsum while achieving a balanced and harmonious appearance.

Neither approach is inherently superior; the best choice depends on the patient's unique anatomy and goals. Some noses are well-suited to preservation, while others require structural modifications for optimal results. The most skilled rhinoplasty surgeons are those who master both techniques and adapt their approach to each individual rather than following a single philosophy. My aim here is not to provide a highly technical analysis but to offer insight into the guiding principles behind these techniques and how they are applied in practice.

A Brief History: Two Parallel Traditions

Preservation rhinoplasty is not a new concept. In the late 19th and early 20th centuries, early surgeons used what were known as push-down and let-down techniques to lower the nasal bridge while keeping it intact. However, as rhinoplasty techniques advanced, structural rhinoplasty became the more widely taught and performed approach for much of the 20th century.

Structural rhinoplasty involves removing excess cartilage and bone to reshape the nose and then rebuilding support with carefully placed grafts. This approach allows for precise control over reshaping and is often the best choice when significant structural changes, correction of asymmetries, or functional improvements are needed.

. . .

While preservation techniques never disappeared, they have gained renewed attention in recent years as refinements in surgical methods have improved their predictability and reliability. Surgeons have revisited and modernized these techniques, incorporating contemporary knowledge of nasal anatomy and healing. Among those who have contributed to this resurgence, Dr. Yves Saban has played a significant role in refining preservation methods and increasing their adoption among rhinoplasty specialists.

Understanding the Differences Between Structural and Preservation Rhinoplasty

Both techniques refine the nose, but they differ in how the nasal bridge is modified and how much of the natural anatomy is maintained.

Structural rhinoplasty involves removing a dorsal hump by shaving down bone and cartilage. This creates an open roof, which requires repositioning the nasal bones and, in many cases, using cartilage grafts to restore support. Because more tissue is removed and rebuilt, recovery can involve more swelling and a longer healing time, but when performed correctly, this approach provides strong, stable, and lasting results.

Preservation rhinoplasty, in contrast, keeps the nasal bridge intact while lowering it from beneath. Rather than cutting directly through the dorsum, precise modifications are made to the structures beneath it, maintaining natural contours while refining the shape. This approach is well-suited to patients whose nasal anatomy allows for adjustments without extensive structural alterations. However, for cases requiring significant reshaping or correction of irregularities, a structural approach or a combination of both methods may be more appropriate.

Ultrasonic Rhinoplasty: Advancing Precision in Both Approaches

One of the most significant advancements in rhinoplasty is the use of ultrasonic technology, also known as Piezo rhinoplasty. This technique uses high-frequency vibrations to sculpt nasal bones with greater precision than traditional methods.

Previously, bone reshaping was performed using chisels or rasps, which, while effective, could sometimes result in unintended fractures. Ultrasonic tools allow for smoother, more controlled modifications while preserving surrounding soft tissue. This technology is not specific to either preservation or structural rhinoplasty but rather serves as a valuable tool that enhances accuracy and minimizes trauma in both approaches.

Choosing the Right Approach

The decision between preservation and structural rhinoplasty is not about favoring one technique over the other, it's about selecting the right method for the patient's individual anatomy, goals, and long-term nasal function. Several factors guide this decision, including the patient's existing nasal structure, the degree of refinement they desire, and the need for long-term stability.

For patients with a dorsal hump who wish to maintain as much of their natural nasal anatomy as possible, preservation techniques may be an excellent option. For those requiring more extensive reshaping, correction of asymmetries, or additional support, a structural approach may be more appropriate. In many cases, elements of both techniques are combined to achieve the best possible result.

Conclusion: The Importance of a Tailored Approach

Rhinoplasty continues to evolve, and no single technique is universally superior. Both preservation and structural methods offer distinct advantages, and the most effective surgeons are those who have mastered both and can apply them as needed.

My approach remains dynamic, guided by each patient's unique anatomy and goals. While the majority of my primary rhinoplasties follow a preservation approach, a significant number still require structural modifications, and the balance between these methods continues to evolve as techniques improve.

CHAPTER 20
MODERN ADVANCES IN RHINOPLASTY: TECHNOLOGY, PRECISION, AND THE FUTURE

Nasal Surgery has always been a delicate balance between art and science. While the fundamental principles of nasal surgery remain the same, technological advancements have dramatically reshaped how surgeons approach the procedure. Precision instruments, digital planning, regenerative medicine, and bioengineered materials have given us tools that enhance results, optimize healing, and minimize trauma—pushing rhinoplasty into an era of unprecedented refinement.

Today, rhinoplasty is no longer about simply removing and reshaping. It's about preserving, refining, and working with each patient's natural anatomy. The introduction of ultrasonic bone sculpting, AI-driven facial analysis, bioengineered cartilage, and regenerative treatments like exosomes and platelet-rich fibrin is revolutionizing the field.

Al thought these advancements don't replace the artistic and technical skills of the surgeon, they allow for greater precision, better healing, and more predictable outcomes. As a surgeon, I'm constantly refining my approach—not just by incorporating these innovations into my own practice but by teaching, researching, and working alongside other experts to push the field forward. Rhinoplasty is always evolving, and these are just a few of the most exciting developments shaping its future.

Ultrasonic Rhinoplasty: Sculpting with Sound Waves
For decades, nasal bone reshaping was done using manual chisels, rasps, and osteotomes—effective tools but ones that relied on force rather than finesse. This traditional approach often resulted in unintentional fractures, asymmetries, and unnecessary trauma to the surrounding soft tissue. It was precise only to a point; beyond that, it was a matter of experience, control, and a little bit of luck.

Ultrasonic rhinoplasty has changed that.

Using high-frequency sound waves, ultrasonic instruments allow surgeons to sculpt nasal bones with extraordinary precision—cutting bone without affecting soft tissue, blood vessels, or cartilage. Instead of breaking the bone manually, this method reshapes it with meticulous control, leading to less swelling, reduced bruising, and a faster, more comfortable recovery.

For patients seeking subtle refinements, ultrasonic rhinoplasty is particularly transformative. The ability to sculpt, rather than fracture, the nasal bridge means fewer irregularities, smoother contours, and a more natural-looking result.

• • •

Ultrasonic technology doesn't replace traditional rhinoplasty techniques, it enhances them, providing a tool that allows for greater control while maintaining the integrity of the nasal framework.

AI and 3D Imaging: The Future of Rhinoplasty Planning

One of the most groundbreaking shifts in modern rhinoplasty is the integration of artificial intelligence and 3D imaging into surgical planning. These technologies are helping surgeons better understand nasal anatomy, facial proportions, and the subtle nuances that define an aesthetically harmonious result.

AI-powered tools can now analyze facial balance, identifying asymmetries and structural proportions with mathematical accuracy. Three-dimensional imaging allows patients to see digital simulations of their potential results, helping them set realistic expectations before surgery.

However, technology is a guide, not a guarantee. No simulation can perfectly predict the final outcome because healing, tissue behavior, and individual anatomy all play a role in how a nose settles over time. While digital imaging provides a roadmap, the artistry of rhinoplasty remains in the hands of the surgeon.

The Promise of Bioengineered Cartilage and 3D Printing

Cartilage grafting has long been a crucial part of rhinoplasty, particularly in cases where additional support is needed. Traditionally, cartilage is harvested from the septum, ear, or rib, but this comes with challenges—additional surgical sites, discomfort, and the risk that the cartilage may warp or resorb over time.

The next frontier? Lab-grown cartilage and 3D printing.
Tissue engineering is paving the way for bioengineered cartilage, which could eliminate the need for donor cartilage altogether. Scientists are now developing custom-shaped grafts grown in controlled environments, designed to mimic the strength and flexibility of natural cartilage while offering a predictable, long-lasting solution.

3D printing is also emerging as a promising innovation in rhinoplasty. In the near future, we may be able to print custom cartilage grafts designed specifically to match each patient's anatomy. This would lead to stronger, more stable grafts, a lower likelihood of warping, and fewer revision surgeries down the line.

Though still in development, these breakthroughs are laying the foundation for a new era of nasal reconstruction, where grafts are no longer limited by the patient's own anatomy but can be designed for optimal function and aesthetics.

A New Era of Rhinoplasty
Rhinoplasty is not what it was a decade ago. What was once thought impossible is now becoming routine, thanks to advancements in precision instruments, digital planning, and regenerative medicine.

· · ·

But innovation doesn't happen in isolation. It requires continuous learning, research, and refinement—a commitment I hold not only in my surgical practice but also in teaching, collaborating, and pushing the boundaries of what's possible.

For those considering rhinoplasty, this is an exciting time. The tools and techniques available today allow for safer procedures, faster recoveries, and more natural-looking results than ever before.

Technology will continue to advance. Our understanding of aesthetics, healing, and regeneration will deepen. And as we embrace these innovations, we will be able to curate a more precise approach to rhinoplasty and produce even more artful and bespoke outcomes.

PART 3: MAKING THE RIGHT CHOICE

CHAPTER 21
TRUE CRAFTSMANSHIP AND THE PURSUIT OF EXCELLENCE

In a world where convenience and speed often take precedence over mastery and excellence, true craftsmanship is becoming a rarity. We live in an era where everything is mass-produced, where efficiency often trumps artistry, and where skill is sometimes sacrificed for accessibility. But there are still those who dedicate their lives to their craft—those who do not seek shortcuts, who do not compromise for the sake of volume, and who hold themselves to a higher standard. These are the artisans, the masters of their field, and when it comes to something as deeply personal and transformative as rhinoplasty, artistry and craftsmanship should be non-negotiable.

Mastery as a Lifelong Pursuit

Mastery is not a title one earns and then rests upon. It is a lifelong pursuit, a relentless dedication to improvement. The Japanese philosophy of **Kaizen**, the idea of continuous refinement, embodies this principle.

. . .

Take the story of Jiro Ono, one of the greatest sushi chefs in the world. Jiro does not simply make sushi—he devotes his life to it. Well into his eighties, he still arrived at his small, Michelin-starred restaurant before dawn, obsessing over every detail. The rice must be at the perfect temperature, the fish sliced with impeccable precision, the balance of flavors refined to perfection. His apprentices spend years mastering the seemingly simple task of cooking rice before they are even allowed to touch the fish. Jiro does not seek speed or efficiency—he seeks mastery. He tastes, adjusts, refines. Even after decades, he never assumes he has learned everything. This is the essence of Kaizen: the relentless pursuit of improvement.

The same philosophy applies to rhinoplasty. A true rhinoplasty surgeon does not operate on autopilot, performing the same procedure in the same way day after day. They refine, evolve, and constantly seek ways to improve. They attend surgical meetings, immerse themselves in the latest advancements, and challenge themselves to question long-held techniques. They do not settle for 'good enough.' They understand that excellence is an ever-moving target.

The Artisan Versus the Mass Producer

Craftsmanship is not just about skill—it's about patience, precision, and an unrelenting commitment to quality. Consider the difference between mass-produced bread and that of a master baker. The supermarket loaf, made for convenience, is churned out in massive quantities, uniform and predictable but flavorless, stale, and lacking character. Meanwhile, the artisan baker arrives at the bakery at four a.m., kneading the dough by hand, allowing it to ferment naturally, carefully controlling the temperature and humidity. Each loaf is a reflection of their expertise and devotion, yielding a depth of flavor and texture that no factory could ever replicate. The difference is unmistakable.

The same principle applies to surgery. Surgery cannot—and should not—be rushed. Rhinoplasty is an operation of millimeters, where even the slightest adjustment can dramatically alter the final outcome. The best surgeons know this and treat the process with the respect it demands. They take their time, meticulously executing every maneuver, checking, adjusting, rechecking, and refining throughout. Every structural modification, every suture, every contouring move is deliberate. There is no room for haste, no place for cutting corners. When a surgeon performs multiple cases in a single day, juggling patient after patient, the time for such meticulous execution simply does not exist. True artisans dedicate themselves fully to each individual case.

A Singular Focus on Excellence

I only operate on one patient per day. It wasn't always this way. Early in my career, I would perform five or six rhinoplasties in a single day. I was proud of that number—I saw it as a mark of skill, of efficiency. And the results were good. But over time, something shifted.

As my experience deepened, so did my obsession with the details. What once seemed like minor nuances became critical elements, each worthy of an extra moment, an extra adjustment. Five cases per day became three. Then two. Now, only one. Because I have learned that rhinoplasty is not a procedure to be rushed. It is not just about executing a series of steps—it is about understanding, adapting, and refining in real time. When performing a primary rhinoplasty, I am done with seventy five percent of the work in the first hour of the operation. The remaining ninety minutes are focused on obsessively refining the twenty five percent that make the difference between good and amazing.

Rhinoplasty is not merely about removing a hump or refining a tip. It's an intricate process of reshaping, restructuring, and restoring balance to the face as a whole. Each patient presents a unique anatomical landscape, a distinct set of challenges and opportunities. The work demands complete focus, absolute precision, and an artist's patience.

The more I operate, the more I realize that the best results come from time—time to evaluate, to adjust, to ensure that every element of the nose blends seamlessly into the patient's features. This is not about efficiency. It's about artistry. And true artistry cannot be rushed.

The Dangers of Routine-Based Surgery

In contrast, there are those who treat surgery as a routine, a checklist to complete rather than a craft to refine. The difference is unmistakable. A mass-producer will approach each nose the same way, applying a formulaic technique that does not account for the patient's individuality. The artisan, however, sees every case as unique, tailoring their approach to enhance what nature has given rather than imposing a one-size-fits-all template.

. . .

There are surgeons who brag about how fast they are. Speed, in itself, is not the enemy—efficiency can be a sign of mastery—but it should never come at the expense of precision, thoughtfulness, and care. The prerequisite is being excellent at your craft first, ensuring that every movement, every adjustment, is deliberate and refined. A surgeon who prioritizes speed over quality risks treating surgery as a mere task rather than a discipline of artistry.

Then there are those who operate by habit, making statements like, *"This is how it's done because that's how I've always done it."* The danger in this mindset is stagnation. A true master never stops evolving. They question their methods, refine their techniques, challenge themselves, and seek out knowledge beyond what they were originally taught. They recognize that mastery is not a destination but a journey of relentless improvement.

The Dedication Beyond the Operating Room
This level of dedication extends beyond the operating room. The true master lives and breathes their craft. They are not simply plastic surgeons; they are sculptors, architects of the human face. Their work is an extension of themselves, a reflection of their passion and commitment. While others may stop learning once they have reached a comfortable level of competence, the master continues to refine, reimagine, and push forward.

Mastery, in any field, requires sacrifice. It demands discipline, patience, and an unyielding pursuit of excellence. There are no shortcuts to true artistry. Rhinoplasty is not an assembly-line procedure; it's a symphony of precision, an orchestration of skill and vision. When choosing a surgeon, the question is not just whether they are trained—it is whether they are devoted. Do they live and breathe their craft? Do they study, improve, and push themselves to higher levels? Do they operate with the meticulous care of an artisan, or the efficiency of a factory line?

The Value of True Artistry

In a world that prioritizes convenience over craftsmanship, finding a surgeon who embodies true artistry is rare but essential. Rhinoplasty is not just about changing a nose; it's about creating balance, harmony, and natural beauty. This level of refinement requires time, dedication, and an unwavering commitment to excellence. Those who take their craft seriously never stop learning, never stop improving, and never settle for mediocrity. When choosing your surgeon, look for the artisan, not the mass producer. Because in the pursuit of true excellence, shortcuts simply do not exist.

CHAPTER 22
STYLE MATTERS

Rhinoplasty isn't just about making a nose smaller, it's about making it more beautiful. More refined, more harmonious, and more suited to the individual face it belongs to. Yet, I constantly see patients focusing only on size reduction, assuming that a smaller nose is automatically an improvement.

I often joke with my patients: *If you take a big potato and make it smaller, it's still a potato.*

A well-executed rhinoplasty is about sculpting. A nose with refined contours, elegant proportions, and a shape that integrates seamlessly with the rest of the face. A nose should never look "done" or like it belongs to someone else. Instead, it should look like it was always meant to be there.

Here's something many patients often don't pay too much

attention to: Your surgeon's personal and surgical style matters.

If you don't like a surgeon's aesthetic, if their results don't resonate with your vision, then no matter how skilled they are, you won't be happy with your outcome.

<u>Finding My Own Style</u>
It took me years to develop and refine my own style. Early in my career, I thought that technical skill alone was enough—that if I mastered the mechanics of rhinoplasty, great results would follow. To a degree, that was true. I learned the techniques, the approaches, the anatomical intricacies. I studied under some of the world's best surgeons, dissected their methods, and replicated their precision.

But something was missing. In my early cases, I would look at my results and think, *Yes, the nose is technically well-executed. The structure is sound. The symmetry is there. But does it actually look...great?*

I wasn't yet seeing that magic—that seamless integration where a nose doesn't just sit on a face but truly belongs there. I realized I was still chasing other surgeons' styles instead of cultivating my own. I had spent so much time perfecting the *how* that I hadn't fully developed my own *why*.

And so, I began the real work—not just of surgery, but of design. I started looking at rhinoplasty as an art form. I studied facial balance, aesthetics, and proportions—not just in medical literature, but in sculpture, photography, and nature. I obsessed over nuances. I analyzed why some noses looked refined while others looked generic, why some results aged gracefully while others didn't.

Over time, I refined my approach, shaping my own style—one that prioritizes elegance, harmony, and balance over simple size reduction. One that adapts to the individual rather than imposing a singular aesthetic on every patient.

As I refined my style, my results transformed. My patients were happier. Their faces looked not just different, but better. More themselves. And that was the moment I knew: style is just as important as skill.

The Pitfall of Choosing a Surgeon without Considering their Style

I see this mistake every day. Patients choosing a surgeon based on name recognition, reputation, or Instagram following rather than whether they actually like the noses that surgeon creates.

Take Mia, for example. She was in her early thirties, well-traveled, well-read, and deeply interested in aesthetics. She came to me frustrated, her voice edged with regret.

"I went to one of the most famous surgeons in the country," she admitted. "His name is everywhere. He's done celebrities, models. I thought if he was good enough for them, he was good enough for me."

. . .

As she talked, it became clear: Mia had never actually liked the noses this surgeon created. She had gone in for the name, assuming that because he was renowned, he could give her what she wanted.

Instead, she ended up with a nose that didn't fit her face. It was too small, too scooped, and the tip looked unnaturally pinched. Technically, the surgery was well done—the incisions were clean, the healing was smooth, and the structure was stable. But when she looked in the mirror, something felt off.

"It's not a bad nose," she said, hesitating. "But it's just… not me."

Mia's story is one I hear all the time. A technically excellent surgeon whose style didn't match the patient's aesthetic will still produce a technically excellent—but fundamentally wrong—nose for that patient.

If the design of your rhinoplasty doesn't align with your face, your personality, and your features, it will never feel right.

Surgeons Have a Style—Make Sure You Like It
Just like fashion designers, architects, and artists, surgeons have a style. Some favor ultra-sculpted looks. Others prefer subtle, barely noticeable refinements. Some lean toward struc-

tured, modelesque noses, while others create softer, more understated changes.

No style is right or wrong, but it has to align with what you want. And before you even consider their surgical style, look at their personal style.

This may sound trivial, but I assure you, it's not. If a surgeon walks into the room in a suit two sizes too big or scrubs that look like they were pulled from the bottom of a laundry pile, take note.

Attention to detail is everything in rhinoplasty. If someone can't be bothered to make sure their own clothes fit, do you really think they're going to obsess over the millimeters that will define your final result?

A surgeon's precision, patience, and attention to detail show up in more ways than just the operating room.

A Matter of Taste: The Brunello Cucinelli Analogy
    If I had to compare rhinoplasty styles to the world of fashion, it's like choosing between different high-end brands.

Take Brunello Cucinelli, for example. His pieces are designed with meticulous craftsmanship, attention to detail, and a refined, understated elegance. There are no flashy logos, no loud patterns; just timeless quality and proportion.

· · ·

Now compare that to Versace—a brand known for bold, high-drama designs. Both are luxury brands, both use the finest materials, but they cater to entirely different aesthetics. If someone walks into a Brunello Cucinelli boutique expecting statement-making fashion, they're going to be disappointed.

The same principle applies to rhinoplasty. If you love hyper-sculpted, ultra-small noses, but you go to a surgeon whose aesthetic leans toward natural, minimal refinements, you're going to end up with a beautifully executed surgery that still doesn't align with what you wanted.

Conversely, if you want a subtle, untouched look but go to a surgeon whose signature is dramatic transformations, you might feel like your nose no longer fits your face. Neither approach is wrong, but the mismatch will leave you unsatisfied.

Final Thoughts: Choose a Surgeon Whose Style You Love
Before booking your surgery, take the time to truly study your surgeon's work.

Look beyond credentials, examine their surgical style. Do their results align with your vision? If you don't love what you see, keep looking. Analyze their outcomes from all angles, not just the side profile. A well-executed nose should look harmonious from the front, three-quarter view, and even from underneath. Most importantly, make sure they can adapt. A great surgeon isn't bound to one aesthetic; they understand how to tailor a nose to complement each patient's unique facial features.

・ ・ ・

Finding my own aesthetic style took years of refinement, trial, and error. I've obsessed over details, studied nuances, and perfected the balance between technical precision and artistic vision. That's what you should expect from your surgeon, not just someone who can perform a procedure, but someone who can craft a result that looks and feels right.

More on choosing your surgeon in next chapter.

CHAPTER 23
WHEN CHOOSING A RHINOPLASTY SURGEON

Choosing a rhinoplasty surgeon is one of the most significant decisions you will ever make. By now you have probably internalized the fact that rhinoplasty is a highly specialized surgery that requires artistic vision, technical precision, and long-term planning. A well-executed rhinoplasty enhances facial harmony, respects a patient's natural features, and maintains or even improves breathing function. Done poorly, it can lead to unnatural results, functional issues, and the need for complex revision surgery.

Yet, with the overwhelming amount of information available, many patients struggle to separate substance from hype. Surgeons can buy followers, pay for awards, and curate an online image that doesn't always reflect their true skill or patient satisfaction. Social media, flashy marketing, and paid accolades can be deceiving, making it harder than ever to make an informed decision. A surgeon's Instagram following, celebrity clientele, or beautifully designed website may be impressive, but none of these things guarantee surgical excellence.

So how do you find the right surgeon? The answer lies in looking beyond the obvious. A surgeon's credentials, reputation, and experience matter, but there's something else that's just as important—your instincts.

Trust Your Gut

For thousands of years, human instincts have helped us assess trustworthiness, competence, and authenticity. That same inner voice—the one that tells you when something feels right or off—is a valuable tool when choosing a surgeon.

Do you feel at ease with them? Do they listen to your concerns, or do they dismiss them? Do they explain things in a way that makes sense to you, or do you leave feeling more confused? Does their demeanor inspire confidence, or do you feel pressured?

Your surgeon should be someone you connect with, someone who makes you feel heard, respected, and understood. If something feels off, trust that feeling. If you find yourself justifying red flags, take a step back. Your gut is often more perceptive than you realize. In my worldview, logic guides, but intuition knows. Trust yours.

Board Certification: A Required Minimum

One of the first things patients check is board certification

—and for good reason. Certification ensures that a surgeon has undergone rigorous training, passed exams, and adheres to professional and ethical standards. But what many don't realize is that board certification is simply the starting point.

Think of it like a driver's license. It proves that a surgeon has met the required standards, understands the fundamentals, and can operate safely. But just as having a driver's license doesn't make someone a racecar driver, board certification alone doesn't tell you much about a surgeon's skill, experience, or aesthetic judgment.

That said, if a surgeon isn't board-certified, that's an immediate red flag. And even within board certification, not all boards are equal. For rhinoplasty, the three most respected boards are:

- **The American Board of Facial Plastic and Reconstructive Surgery (ABFPRS)** – This certifies surgeons specializing exclusively in facial plastic surgery, including rhinoplasty.
- **The American Board of Plastic Surgery (ABPS)** – This certifies surgeons trained in plastic and reconstructive surgery of the entire body, including the face.
- **The American Board of Otolaryngology – Head and Neck Surgery (ABOTO-HNS)** – This certifies surgeons who specialize in ear, nose, and throat (ENT) surgery, including nasal surgery and rhinoplasty.

If a surgeon claims to be "board-certified" but it's not through one of these boards, it's worth investigating further.

Do They Specialize in Rhinoplasty?

Many plastic surgeons perform rhinoplasty, but not all of them specialize in it. Specialization does not mean rhinoplasty is *all* they do. It means they take a special interest in rhinoplasty and keep up with its advancements, and perform a high number of it. Are there plastic surgeons out there who can perform all procedures at the highest level? Perhaps, but I have not yet met one. Rhinoplasty is one of the most technically demanding surgeries in plastic surgery, requiring an in-depth understanding of nasal anatomy, function, and aesthetics. A surgeon who primarily focuses on body procedures but occasionally does rhinoplasty may not have the same level of expertise as someone who dedicates most of their practice to it.

If you're seeking a revision, ethnic rhinoplasty, or complex structural work, it's even more critical to find a surgeon with significant experience in those areas. Not all rhinoplasties are the same, and different techniques require different expertise.

How Their Team Feels About Them Matters

A great surgeon isn't just respected by their peers, they're respected by the people who work with them every day. Surgical staff often have a unique perspective on a surgeon's abilities. They see their work up close, day in and day out, and understand not just their technical skill, but also their ethics, integrity, and consistency.

One of the most revealing questions you can ask a surgeon's team is:

"Would you trust this surgeon to operate on your nose?"

The way a staff member responds—whether with enthusiasm or hesitation—can be incredibly telling. If they wouldn't trust the surgeon with their own face, why should you?

Surgical Environment: Where and How They Operate

Not all surgical environments are the same. Some surgeons operate in third-party surgery centers where they have little control over the nursing staff, anesthesia providers, or surgical instruments. In these settings, anesthesia providers are randomly assigned, which means they may not be familiar with the surgeon's specific protocols or the level of finesse required for rhinoplasty.

If your surgeon operates in an accredited facility, it's a positive sign. Accreditation ensures that the operating room meets the highest standards of safety, equipment, and emergency preparedness. Some of the most reputable accreditation organizations include:

- AAAASF (American Association for Accreditation of Ambulatory Surgery Facilities)
- JCAHO (Joint Commission on Accreditation of Healthcare Organizations)
- AAAHC (Accreditation Association for Ambulatory Health Care)

If a surgeon operates in a facility without accreditation, it's worth asking why.

Cost Transparency: What's Included?

A reputable surgeon provides clear, upfront pricing. Some practices offer all-inclusive pricing, while others itemize fees, which can lead to unexpected costs. Understanding what is and isn't included can prevent surprises down the road.

Questions to ask include:

- Are operating room and anesthesia fees included, or separate?
- What's covered in post-operative care? Are follow-up treatments like laser therapy or scar management included?
- Does the surgeon have a structured approach to revisions if needed?

While cost is an important factor, it should never be the sole deciding factor. The lowest price may not always be the best value, and an unusually low fee could be a red flag.

Final Thoughts
To find the right rhinoplasty surgeon one must look beyond mere popularity and fame. The decision must be grounded in the trifecta of outstanding credentials and technical mastery, surgical and aesthetic style, and your connection with the surgical team and your gut feeling.

Ask the tough questions. Look at long-term results, not just early post-op photos. Pay attention to how they communicate and whether they truly listen. Most importantly, trust your instincts. Your face is not a trend. This is a decision that will impact you for the rest of your life. Take your time, do your research, and choose wisely.

CHAPTER 24
HOW TO ASSESS BEFORE-AND-AFTER PHOTOS CRITICALLY

Before-and-after photos are one of the most useful tools for evaluating a rhinoplasty surgeon's work. They provide a tangible way to assess a surgeon's aesthetic style, their approach to nasal refinement, and the quality of their results. However, while these images can be incredibly informative, they should also be viewed with a discerning eye. Photography techniques, lighting, angles, and even the timing of the photos can all influence how a result appears.

The goal of this chapter is not to cast doubt on before-and-after photos but to help patients analyze them more objectively—noticing details that go beyond the initial impact of a striking transformation.

The Role of Photography in Surgical Results

Photography plays a crucial role in documenting rhinoplasty outcomes, but like any visual medium, it comes with variables that can subtly influence perception. Some of these differences are unintentional, while others can make results appear more dramatic than they truly are.

Lighting can significantly impact how a nose looks. Strong overhead lighting in a "before" photo may cast shadows that exaggerate irregularities, while soft, even lighting in an "after" photo can create a smoother, more refined appearance. Lens distortion is another factor—some "before" photos are taken with a wide-angle lens that makes the nose look larger or more projected, while "after" photos may be captured with a more neutral lens, making the difference seem more pronounced.

Camera position and zoom can also influence perception. A "before" photo taken up close and an "after" photo taken slightly farther away can make the nose appear smaller or more proportional, even if the surgical change is subtle. Additionally, makeup, facial expression, and skin tone can play a role. Many "before" photos are taken with patients completely bare-faced, while "after" photos may include foundation or contouring that enhances the definition of the nose. A more relaxed expression in the "after" shot can also contribute to an overall sense of facial harmony.

Finally, digital retouching—while uncommon among reputable surgeons—can be a factor. Some images may undergo minor adjustments, such as skin smoothing, lighting corrections, or contrast changes, unintentionally enhancing the post-surgical look. However, a great surgeon doesn't need to manipulate their work. Their results should speak for themselves.

· · ·

The Importance of Long-Term Results

When evaluating before-and-after photos, it's important to look beyond immediate post-operative images. While intraoperative photos taken on the operating table can showcase technical precision, they don't reveal how a nose will evolve over time. Swelling, tissue settling, and scar maturation all influence the final outcome, which takes months or even years to fully develop.

When reviewing a surgeon's work, pay attention to whether there are consistent follow-up images at six months, one year, or longer. Do the results remain refined over time, or do they only look good in the immediate post-op phase? A well-structured nose should maintain its shape rather than collapsing or shifting as the healing process unfolds.

A skilled rhinoplasty surgeon doesn't just create an aesthetically pleasing result for the first few months, they ensure that the nose ages gracefully, preserving both its integrity and function long after surgery.

Recognizing a Surgeon's Style

Every great surgeon has an aesthetic signature—a unique approach to refinement, balance, and proportion. While consistency is a positive sign, it's equally important that each result looks natural to the individual patient rather than following a uniform template.

When reviewing before-and-after photos, look for variation. Do all the noses look identical, or does each one complement the patient's unique facial features? A skilled surgeon should have experience with different nasal types, including a range of ethnic backgrounds and structural variations. The best results are elegant and timeless, not overly stylized to match fleeting trends.

Rhinoplasty should never be a "one-size-fits-all" procedure. A well-executed surgery enhances a patient's natural beauty, respects their facial proportions, and preserves their unique identity.

Final Thoughts: Looking Beyond the Image

Before-and-after photos are an invaluable tool, but they should not be the only factor in choosing a surgeon. A well-trained eye can recognize the difference between a well-done rhinoplasty and an image that has been influenced by external factors. Patients should seek consistency, authenticity, and long-term stability when assessing results.

Ultimately, the best rhinoplasty surgeons take great pride in their work, and their results stand the test of time. By approaching before-and-after photos with a critical but fair mindset, patients can gain a deeper understanding of a surgeon's artistry and skill—ensuring that their decision is based on more than just a single striking transformation.

CHAPTER 25
THE SETTING MATTERS AS MUCH AS THE SURGEON

When people think about rhinoplasty, they focus almost entirely on choosing the right surgeon—reviewing credentials, before-and-after photos, and patient testimonials. But one factor that's just as important, and often overlooked, is where the surgery takes place and who is in the room. These elements don't just shape the experience; they influence the outcome in ways most patients never realize.

For years, I operated in hospitals and outpatient surgery centers. I did everything I could to control the experience—bringing my own anesthesiologist, carefully transporting my custom instruments, arriving hours early to ensure everything was properly sterilized. But no matter how much effort I put in, there were always variables I couldn't control.

The Hospital Experience: Not Necessarily Designed for Rhinoplasty

In a hospital setting, you're one of many patients. You

check in alongside people undergoing all kinds of procedures, from orthopedic surgeries to emergency cases. Privacy is limited. Your case might be delayed or even rescheduled if a more urgent case needs the operating room. The staff working with you—the nurses, anesthesiologists, and surgical assistants—are different every time. Hospitals prioritize high-risk cases like neurosurgery, cardiac surgery, and trauma, meaning the team assigned to your rhinoplasty might not have much experience with facial plastic surgery.

Beyond the people in the room, the tools and materials hospitals use are chosen for efficiency and cost-saving rather than precision or optimal healing. The instruments are often standard-issue, designed for general surgeries, not the delicate refinements of rhinoplasty. The sutures are whatever bulk brand the facility has stocked—not necessarily the finest, longest-lasting materials for delicate nasal structures. Anesthesia medications are determined by hospital-wide protocols, not necessarily selected to minimize swelling and ensure the smoothest recovery.

Even after surgery, the experience remains unpredictable. Who monitors your recovery? It might be someone familiar with facial surgery or someone who's never handled a rhinoplasty patient before. In hospitals and surgery centers, post-op care is handled by whoever is on shift. They may not know your procedure's nuances, and their goal is to move patients through efficiently rather than provide individualized attention.

Ironically, despite all these limitations, having surgery at a hospital or outpatient surgery center is often far more expensive. Facility fees, anesthesia costs, and hidden upcharges quickly add up. Many patients assume that because hospitals are large institutions, they must offer the highest level of care, but in reality, rhinoplasty in a hospital is often more expensive and less tailored to the patient's needs.

Surgery Centers: Not All Are the Same

It's worth noting that not all surgery centers are like this. There are some very well-run, aesthetically focused surgery centers designed specifically for plastic surgery patients. These facilities often offer a better experience than hospitals—more privacy, fewer delays, and staff who are accustomed to working with aesthetic patients. However, the biggest limitation of surgery centers, even the very good ones, is that in many cases surgeons do not own or control them. Someone else calls the shots. The facility is still managed by a separate entity, which means surgeons don't always have control over the staff, the equipment, the scheduling, or even the quality of the materials used.

One day, a surgeon may have an excellent anesthesiologist and a highly skilled surgical tech assisting them. The next time, they may not. The ability to evolve and fine-tune processes as a team is limited when the staff is constantly changing, and decisions about the operating environment are made by administrators rather than the surgeon.

Why Every Detail Matters

I realized over time that having control over every detail is just as important as the surgery itself. Rhinoplasty is an intricate, highly individualized procedure—it cannot be approached with a one-size-fits-all mentality. That's why I made the decision to create my own fully purpose-built surgical microcosm.

Everything we use is state-of-the-art and selected for quality, precision, and patient comfort. The instruments in my hands are not generic—they are custom-made for the exact techniques I use, designed for precision work. The sutures are the highest quality available, carefully selected to minimize scarring and ensure the strongest, longest-lasting results. The anesthesia medications are tailored for facial surgery, chosen to ensure a smooth experience, minimal swelling, and the fastest possible recovery.

Beyond the tools, the team matters just as much. My anesthesiologist is not someone randomly assigned to the case. He is someone I have worked with for years, who specializes in facial surgery, and who understands exactly how to tailor anesthesia to minimize discomfort and optimize results. My surgical assistants are not a rotating group of nurses who have never worked with me before, they are highly trained professionals who know our protocols inside and out, ensuring that every procedure flows seamlessly. Can't you tell we proud?

This level of control is also why I always have to decline requests to operate in other cities and countries. While I'm honored by the trust these patients place in me, so much of what makes this process successful depends on the team, the tools, and the controlled environment we've created. A surgeon's skill is only one piece of the puzzle—the instruments, the anesthesia, the sutures, and the experience of the team all greatly contribute to the final outcome.

The Difference in Experience

When every element is optimized the overall experience is better. You are not one of many. You're not shuffled from one department to another, seeing a different face at every stage of the process. The same people who meet you at your consultation are with you on surgery day and throughout your recovery. There is no rushed handoff. No wondering who will be putting you to sleep for the procedure or who will be taking care of you post-op. This kind of personalized care is what *should* be the standard in aesthetic medicine.

CHAPTER 26
THE FINANCIAL ASPECT OF RHINOPLASTY: PRICE, COST, VALUE

One of the first questions patients ask when considering rhinoplasty is, *"How much does it cost?"* It's a fair question. Rhinoplasty is a significant financial investment—often one of the most substantial personal expenses someone considers. But there's an even more important question that many forget to ask:

"What does that price actually include?"

Rhinoplasty costs vary widely. Some quotes seem steep, while others look like a bargain. But price alone doesn't tell the whole story. To compare quotes fairly, it really comes down to what it is exactly you're paying for. Let's take a closer look.

The Real Cost of a Bargain – Emily's Story

Emily had wanted a rhinoplasty for years. She was thoughtful, well-researched, and knew exactly what she wanted—something refined and natural, nothing extreme, just a nose that suited her face.

She loved my work but hesitated when we discussed the cost. *"I have another consultation with a surgeon who quoted me several thousand dollars less. I just don't know if I can justify the higher price,"* she told me.

I understood her hesitation. Rhinoplasty is a major financial decision, and the cost isn't insignificant. After our consultation, she took her time to consider her options and ultimately decided to go with the lower-cost provider.

Two years later, she walked back into my office—this time not with excitement, but with regret. Her nose was too small for her face, lacked definition, and worst, she was struggling to breathe.

She explained how, at the time, she had assumed that any aesthetic surgeon could perform a rhinoplasty. She had convinced herself that as long as a doctor specialized in cosmetic procedures, they could reshape a nose just as well as anything or anyone else. She had focused on the end goal—getting the nose she had always dreamed of—without fully understanding the process or what truly mattered in a rhinoplasty surgeon; a mistake I see all too often.

When surgery day arrived, she was filled with anticipation, imagining the fresh start ahead. But when the cast came off, her stomach dropped. Something was off. The nose in the mirror wasn't what she had envisioned. It looked crooked, undefined, and completely out of sync with her face.

• • •

Her surgeon reassured her that it was just swelling, something that would resolve over time. But deep down, she knew. This wasn't just swelling. This wasn't what she had wanted.

Months passed, and the issues became even more obvious. The asymmetry remained, the structure felt weak, and more than anything, it simply didn't enhance her face the way she had imagined. That's when she realized what she had overlooked—not all rhinoplasty is created equal.

"I focused so much on price," she admitted, shaking her head. *"I should have been looking at skill and results."*

Now, she had to do it all over again. And this time, it would cost her far more—financially, emotionally, and physically—than if she had simply chosen the right surgeon the first time.

Her story isn't unique. A few years ago, we ran the numbers and found that over 18% of patients who initially chose another surgeon solely based on financial reasons, eventually return to me for a revision. That number is probably higher in reality as many of them likely go somewhere else for their revision. That's a costly mistake in every sense of the word.

Why Rhinoplasty Costs Vary

Rhinoplasty pricing depends on several factors—location, surgeon experience, and whether fees are bundled or separate. Some quotes include everything from anesthesia to post-op care, while others appear lower at first glance but leave out key expenses that add up later.

A lower-cost quote might include only the surgeon's fee, while additional charges for the operating room, anesthesia, and post-op care are billed separately. The type of facility also matters. A fully accredited surgical center with modern safety protocols costs more to maintain than a standard outpatient clinic, but it also ensures a higher level of care.

Anesthesia is another factor. Some practices work with board-certified anesthesiologists, while others cut costs by using nurse anesthetists or general physicians for sedation. While legal, this difference in expertise can impact the safety and comfort of the procedure.

Postoperative care is often overlooked, but it plays a major role in recovery and final results. Some practices include multiple follow-ups, taping, scar management, and laser treatments, while others charge extra or offer minimal support beyond the first post-op visit. Patients often assume all surgeons will be equally available for follow-ups, but in some cases, communication is primarily handled by office staff, limiting direct access to the surgeon.

A comprehensive price doesn't just reflect the surgery itself, it reflects the entire experience, from A to Z.

Cutting Costs vs. Cutting Corners

Some surgeons offer lower pricing not necessarily because

they are less skilled, but because they reduce overhead in ways that affect the patient's experience and final result.

Lower-cost clinics may use older anesthetic drugs, which can increase post-op nausea and grogginess. They may rely on traditional surgical tools instead of advanced ultrasonic technology, requiring more manual force for bone reshaping, which can lead to greater swelling and bruising. Some reduce costs by using non-board-certified anesthesiologists, a legal but significant difference in patient care.

Post-op care is another area where costs are sometimes trimmed. Some practices limit follow-up visits or don't include additional healing treatments like lymphatic massage, scar management, or LED light therapy, all of which can improve recovery and final results.

While none of these factors alone determine the outcome of a rhinoplasty, together they contribute to the overall level of care. The difference isn't just in the final result but in the entire journey—comfort during surgery, safety during recovery, and the confidence of knowing you're in expert hands.

Making Rhinoplasty More Accessible

Many patients assume that if they don't have the full cost saved up, they can't move forward with surgery. But just like education, a home, or medical care, rhinoplasty is an investment—and it doesn't always have to be paid all at once.

. . .

There are financing options that can make surgery more accessible. Medical credit plans like CareCredit, Patient Fi and Alphaeon offer low-interest financing, while some practices allow patients to pay in installments before surgery. Banks and credit unions also offer personal loans for elective procedures.

Many people use financing for major life investments—it's worth exploring what options exist for surgical care.

Final Thoughts

When considering rhinoplasty, it's important to look beyond the price tag and ask deeper questions. What is included in the total cost? What level of safety and postoperative care is provided? Does the surgeon's work reflect the aesthetic you're looking for?

There's no universal "right" decision, only the decision that's right for you. By understanding the true costs involved, you can make a choice that aligns with your goals, budget, and expectations. Wait until you're ready, and go with a decision that sits right with your heart. Your face is no place for bargain shopping.

CHAPTER 27
NAVIGATING THE REALITIES OF MEDICAL TOURISM

The appeal is undeniable. A "luxury" surgical experience abroad, often at a fraction of the cost, complete with five-star accommodations and the promise of a quick, seamless transformation. It's easy to see why more and more patients are choosing to travel for rhinoplasty.

And let me be clear: exceptional rhinoplasty surgeons can be found all over the world. Some of the most skilled, ethical, and talented surgeons I know—mentors, colleagues, and friends I deeply respect—practice outside the U.S. At the same time, I've seen firsthand the devastating consequences of choosing a surgeon based solely on price or location.

The truth is, neither the U.S. nor any other country has a monopoly on great (or poor) surgeons. A country's reputation doesn't guarantee a surgeon's expertise. What matters is not *where* a surgeon is based, but *who* they are—their skill set, experience, surgical philosophy, and ability to deliver safe, long-term results.

Over the years, I have met hundreds of patients who deeply regretted their decision to have surgery abroad. Some sought me out because they had no access to follow-up care. Others came in desperation, their noses collapsing, their breathing compromised, their faces permanently altered by aggressive or poorly executed techniques.

If you're considering traveling for rhinoplasty, you need to understand the full picture. The biggest risks aren't just about the surgeon—it's about the entire system surrounding the procedure.

- What happens if something goes wrong?
- Who is responsible for your care once you leave?
- Who is ensuring the quality of your anesthesia and postoperative treatment?

This isn't about fear, it's about informed decision-making. Your face, your breathing, and your long-term health deserve nothing less than the full truth.

The Illusion of Immediate Post-Op Perfection

One of the most common things I hear from patients who had surgery abroad is: *"But my nose looked amazing right after surgery!"*

. . .

They pull up post-op photos from the clinic, images that seem to showcase a sleek, straight, and refined nose. Then I look at them in real time, months later—and the nose in front of me tells a completely different story. Granted there is a selection bias here: Patients who are happy with their results do not need to come see me, so I only end up seeing those who are experiencing problems.

Swelling can temporarily disguise surgical flaws. A nose may appear flawless in the first few weeks, only to reveal deep structural problems as the swelling subsides. Taping and compression dressings can hold the nose in an artificially ideal position, creating a misleading sense of symmetry and definition. And in some cases, post-op images are subtly enhanced, edited, or carefully lit to create an illusion of perfection; not to mention the nose will undergo fibrotic changes overtime, too.

Although many of the most reputable and skilled surgeons I know abroad offer their patients low-cost or free revision surgery, this is not the case for all. By the time the real results settle in, the patient is thousands of miles away, unable to return for adjustments or corrections. That's when reality sets in.

Sarah's Story: The Nose That Collapsed
Sarah had dreamed of a rhinoplasty for years. She spent months researching, scrolling through before-and-after galleries, and finally found a clinic that promised everything she wanted—at a price that seemed too good to pass up.

· · ·

For the first few weeks after surgery, she was thrilled. The photos from her clinic looked perfect. But slowly, everything started falling apart.

Her nasal tip, once defined, collapsed so dramatically that it nearly touched her upper lip when she smiled. The bridge, once smooth, buckled inward, leaving an unnatural indentation. One nostril was now significantly larger than the other, and worst of all, she could no longer breathe properly through her nose.

When I examined her during our consultation, it became clear that the structure of her nose had been compromised. The cartilage had been shaved down aggressively, leaving it with no ability to maintain its shape. Inside, her nasal lining was suffocated by scar tissue, restricting airflow.

During revision surgery, I had to rebuild her nose from the ground up. Using rib cartilage, I reconstructed the framework, restored proper support, and opened her airway. It was an intricate, complex operation—far more difficult and involved than her original rhinoplasty ever would have been.

Her biggest regret? Focusing only on how her nose looked in those first few weeks, rather than whether it had been built to last.

The Unseen Risks of Anesthesia: Who Is Putting You to Sleep?

Most patients spend hours researching their surgeon, but very few think to ask about the anesthesia team. Yet anesthesia is one of the most critical—and potentially life-threatening—parts of any surgery.

- Who is administering your anesthesia?
- What medications are being used?
- What safety protocols are in place?
- How is your airway being managed during the procedure?

In my practice, I work exclusively with board-certified anesthesiologists who specialize in facial surgery. These are professionals I know, trust, and collaborate with regularly. Our protocols are strict, our medications are carefully selected, and our emergency response plans are well-rehearsed.

In many medical tourism settings, these same assurances don't always exist. Some clinics use non-specialized anesthetists to reduce costs, and the drugs and equipment used may not always adhere to the same regulatory standards. If something goes wrong under anesthesia, who is there to ensure your safety?

Rhinoplasty is an elective procedure, but anesthesia is life or death. It deserves just as much scrutiny as the surgeon performing your operation.

Julia's Story: The Nose That Vanished

Julia's rhinoplasty abroad seemed to go smoothly at first. But six months later, she noticed something alarming.

Her nostrils collapsed inward every time she inhaled. The tip of her nose seemed to be sinking into her face. The bridge, once defined, was now so over-reduced that it barely looked like she had a nose at all.

When she reached out to the clinic, she was reassured by the "clinic assistant" that this was normal; she just needed to "wait for the swelling to subside." But this wasn't swelling, this was structural failure.

Her original procedure had been designed to make her nose smaller and improve her breathing. During our consultation, I immediately noticed that her bridge had been over-resected, and her nose had no support left. To correct the collapse, I had to take the nose entirely apart, reconstruct her nasal valves, and to my surprise, the septum had not even been touched and remained deviated- which we of course corrected. What should have been a straightforward procedure had now become a highly complex, invasive revision.

Her biggest regret? Not realizing that once something went wrong, she had no one to turn to.

The Question No One Asks: Who Is Accountable?

One of the most crucial questions any patient should ask before traveling for surgery is: *What happens if something goes wrong?*

• • •

In countries with strict medical oversight, surgeons are held accountable by licensing boards, malpractice laws, and professional ethics committees. If a patient experiences negligence or malpractice, they have legal recourse.

But when you travel for surgery, those safeguards may not always exist.

If you wake up with unexpected complications, who is responsible? If your results don't match what was promised, what are your options? If you suffer permanent damage, who do you turn to for help?

Many medical tourism clinics cater to international patients precisely because they know legal recourse is difficult. Some patients have tried reaching their original clinic for help, only to be met with silence—emails unanswered, messages ignored, even phone numbers blocked.

If you're considering rhinoplasty abroad, ask yourself: *Am I comfortable knowing that if something goes wrong, I may have no way to fix it?*

I've seen too many patients walk into my office in distress, their dream of a perfect nose turned into a nightmare of breathing difficulties, collapsing structure, and irreversible regret. Your first rhinoplasty is the most important one. If done correctly, it should last a lifetime. If done poorly, it can lead to years of additional surgeries, emotional distress, and permanent complications.

This isn't to say that all surgery abroad is bad. There are extraordinary surgeons across the world, and I have nothing but respect for my colleagues who uphold the highest standards of care. But not every surgeon does that and you need to make sure you do you due diligence and research. If you're considering aesthetic surgery abroad, you need to be meticulous.

Know who your surgeon is. Know who your anesthesiologist is. Know who will be there for you if something goes wrong.

CHAPTER 28

COMMON MYTHS ABOUT RHINOPLASTY: SEPARATING FACT FROM FICTION

Throughout this book, we've explored the many aspects of rhinoplasty—its history, techniques, the intricacies of nasal anatomy, and what makes a successful outcome. By now, it should be clear that rhinoplasty is far more than just a cosmetic procedure. It's a blend of art, science, and surgical precision, requiring an in-depth understanding of both form and function.

Yet, despite all the advancements in the field, myths about rhinoplasty persist. Misinformation spreads easily, whether through social media, outdated medical advice, or unrealistic portrayals in entertainment. Some misconceptions make people hesitant about the procedure, while others create false expectations that lead to disappointment.

In this chapter, we'll tackle some of the most common myths surrounding rhinoplasty and set the record straight.

. . .

Myth #1: Rhinoplasty is Only About Aesthetics

A common misconception is that rhinoplasty is purely a cosmetic procedure performed only to enhance appearance. While improving the shape of the nose is often part of the goal, rhinoplasty is frequently performed to correct functional issues, such as breathing difficulties caused by a deviated septum, nasal valve collapse, or previous trauma.

A well-done rhinoplasty doesn't just refine how a nose looks, it ensures the airway remains open and stable for life. No surgical result can be considered successful if it compromises nasal function.

Myth #2: You Can Bring a Photo and Get That Exact Nose

It's normal for patients to bring in inspiration photos to help convey their aesthetic preferences, but noses are not interchangeable. A nose that looks perfect on one person may not complement another's unique facial structure. The key to a successful rhinoplasty is creating harmony between the nose and the rest of the face, not simply copying someone else's features.

Surgeons take into account factors like bone structure, skin thickness, and overall facial proportions when designing a patient's rhinoplasty.

Myth #3: The Smaller the Nose, the Better the Result

There's a misconception that a smaller nose automatically looks more refined or attractive. In reality, over-reducing the nose can lead to long-term structural issues, including nasal collapse, difficulty breathing, and an unnatural or infantile appearance.

In my view, rhinoplasty is about achieving the right balance for each individual's face. Removing too much support from the nasal framework can weaken the structure over time, leading to a pinched or collapsed look. A well-executed rhinoplasty refines and reshapes while preserving the integrity and function of the nose.

Myth #4: Any Aesthetic Surgeon Can Perform Rhinoplasty
Not all plastic surgeons specialize in rhinoplasty. This procedure is one of the most complex in the field of aesthetic surgery, requiring a deep understanding of nasal anatomy, structural support, and aesthetic refinement. A surgeon who primarily focuses on body procedures may not have the same level of expertise as one who specializes in facial surgery.

Choosing a surgeon with extensive experience in rhinoplasty —particularly one who has dedicated their career to the nuances of nasal surgery—can make the difference between a seamless, natural-looking result and an average formless nose- or worse, the need for a difficult revision later.

Myth #5: Rhinoplasty Always Looks Obvious
Some people hesitate to get rhinoplasty because they fear they'll end up with an unnatural, "plastic" look. This stereotype comes from poorly executed surgeries, where noses are made too small, over-scooped, or stripped of their natural structure.

• • •

A well-done rhinoplasty should be nearly undetectable. It enhances facial balance without drawing attention. People should notice that you look refreshed, but they shouldn't be able to pinpoint why. A good rhinoplasty looks as if it belongs on your face, not like something that was added or altered.

Myth #6: The Results are Instant
Rhinoplasty is a process, not an overnight transformation. Swelling, tissue healing, and structural settling all take time. While changes will be visible as soon as the cast comes off, the final result unfolds gradually over several months, sometimes up to a year.

The tip of the nose, in particular, takes the longest to refine. Patience is crucial, as minor asymmetries or swelling fluctuations in the early months do not necessarily reflect the final outcome.

Myth #7: Rhinoplasty is Painful
Pain is one of the biggest concerns for those considering surgery, but rhinoplasty is not a painful procedure. Most patients describe the discomfort as mild to moderate, similar to congestion from a bad cold. Modern techniques, along with proper post-operative care, make recovery much smoother than many expect. Of course, everyone's pain tolerance is different but the majority of my patients tell me a few Tylenols the first few days was all they needed.

Myth #8: Only Women Get Rhinoplasty
Rhinoplasty is not gender-specific. Men seek rhinoplasty

for the same reasons as women—whether to improve breathing, correct a structural issue, or enhance facial balance. The approach for male rhinoplasty often differs to preserve masculine features, but the goal remains the same: a natural, well-proportioned nose that fits the face.

Myth #9: Anesthesia Used in Rhinoplasty is Dangerous

All surgeries carry some level of risk, but modern anesthesia is extremely safe. The anesthetic techniques used in rhinoplasty are well-studied and have an excellent safety record, even for high-risk patients. In my practice we use an anesthesia type called Total Intravenous Anesthesia-or TIVA- which is considered safer and easier on the patients. With correct preoperative testing and clearance and being under the care of an experienced board-certified anesthesiologist helps ensure that the procedure is safe and comfortable.

Myth #10: Rhinoplasty Leaves Visible Scars

Concerns about scarring are understandable, but rhinoplasty incisions are typically very small and strategically placed. In a closed rhinoplasty, all incisions are inside the nostrils, leaving no external scars. Even in an open rhinoplasty, where a small incision is made under the columella, the scar is almost invisible once healed.

Myth #11: Rhinoplasty is Only for the Wealthy

The idea that rhinoplasty is only for celebrities or the ultra-wealthy is outdated. While it is an investment, many patients come from all walks of life and choose to undergo surgery for personal or medical reasons. Financing options and payment plans make the procedure accessible to a broader range of people.

· · ·

Myth #12: Your Mindset has No Effect on the Outcome
The mental aspect of surgery is just as important as the physical one. Patients who approach rhinoplasty with realistic expectations, patience, and trust in the process tend to have better experiences. Those who fixate on every minor change, stress over early healing fluctuations, or constantly compare their progress to others often struggle more during recovery.

A confident, relaxed mindset allows for a smoother journey, both physically and emotionally. Trusting the process is key to achieving the best possible result.

Final Thoughts
So far in this book, we've learned a great deal about rhinoplasty—its complexities, the surgical process, and what makes a successful outcome. This chapter has addressed some of the most common misconceptions, but this is by no means a comprehensive list. New myths emerge all the time, shaped by trends, misinformation, and unrealistic portrayals of plastic surgery.

The most important takeaway is this: rhinoplasty is not just about making a nose smaller or following beauty trends. It's about balance, function, and long-term harmony with the rest of the face. The best results come from choosing the right surgeon, setting realistic expectations, and understanding that rhinoplasty is a process, not a quick fix.

CHAPTER 29
HOW TO TALK TO FAMILY AND FRIENDS ABOUT YOUR DECISION

Deciding to undergo rhinoplasty is a deeply personal choice, often made after years of consideration. But while you may feel ready, sharing this decision with family and friends can be a different kind of challenge. Even those who love and support you might have opinions—some encouraging, others skeptical, and a few outright dismissive. These reactions can feel confusing or even frustrating, but they usually come from a place of care, curiosity, or misunderstanding rather than judgment.

The key to navigating these conversations is to approach them with **clarity, patience, and confidence** while also allowing space for your loved ones to process your decision.

Why People React Differently

People's responses to cosmetic surgery are often shaped by their own beliefs, cultural influences, or personal experiences. Some will trust your judgment without hesitation, offering words of support and encouragement. Others may express concern, not because they doubt your decision, but because they want to be sure you've thought it through. Questions like *"Are you sure you need this?"* or *"What if you don't like it?"* often come from a place of love, even if they feel unsettling in the moment.

Parents and partners, in particular, may struggle with the idea of change. A mother might say, *"But I love your nose just the way it is,"* not realizing that her attachment to your appearance doesn't necessarily reflect how you feel about it. A spouse might worry, *"Will you still look like you?"* because they associate your features with your identity. These concerns are natural and don't mean they disapprove—they simply need reassurance that your decision is about enhancing, not erasing, who you are.

Then there are those who respond with skepticism or outright dismissal. Comments like *"Why would you do that?"* or *"You should just learn to love yourself"* can feel invalidating, but they often come from a place of misunderstanding rather than malice. Many people don't realize that rhinoplasty isn't about vanity or insecurity, it's about harmony, confidence, and feeling like the best version of yourself.

How to Introduce the Conversation

How you present your decision can shape how others respond. If you bring it up hesitantly or as if you're seeking permission, you may invite more unsolicited advice. Instead, **speak with** calm confidence and make it clear that this is something you've thought through.

• • •

A straightforward approach often works best: *"I've been considering rhinoplasty for a long time, and I've decided to move forward with it. I feel confident in my decision and wanted to share it with you."*

If someone expresses concern, acknowledge their feelings while reassuring them that you've done your research: *"I understand why you're asking, and I appreciate you looking out for me. I've put a lot of thought into this, and I trust my surgeon completely."*

Some may ask why you want the procedure at all. In those cases, keeping your explanation simple and personal is often enough: *"It's something I've always wanted, and I know it will help me feel more comfortable in my own skin."* There's no need to justify or defend your choice beyond what feels right to you.

Navigating Concerns from Loved Ones

Close family members, especially parents and spouses, may need more time to come around. Their concern isn't necessarily about the surgery itself, it's about wanting the best for you. If they worry about safety, let them know you've chosen an experienced, qualified surgeon. If they fear you'll regret it, reassure them that this is not an impulsive choice but one you've considered deeply.

Sometimes, they simply need to hear that you'll still look like *you*. Letting them know that rhinoplasty, when done correctly, enhances rather than drastically changes your features can put their minds at ease.

・・・

In cases where someone is persistently negative or dismissive, it's okay to set boundaries. A gentle but firm response like *"I understand that you may not agree, but this is something I've chosen for myself, and I'd appreciate your support"* can help close the conversation without escalating tension.

Deciding Who to Tell
Not everyone needs to know about your decision. Some people choose to share only with those closest to them, while others are more open. If you anticipate judgment or criticism from certain individuals, you may decide to wait until after the procedure or not mention it at all.

Similarly, if privacy is important to you, you are under no obligation to explain your decision to coworkers, acquaintances, or anyone outside your trusted circle. Your choice is yours alone, and you get to decide how much or how little you share.

Confidence in Your Choice
At the heart of these conversations is a simple truth: this is your face, your body, and your decision. While it's natural to want support from those closest to you, it's equally important to remember that their opinions do not define your choice.

Approaching these discussions with confidence and reassurance can help ease concerns, but not everyone will understand, and that's okay. The most important thing is that you feel at peace with your decision, knowing it's something you are doing for yourself and no one else.

CHAPTER 30
TRUSTING THE PROCESS IS KEY

One of the most important things I've observed repeatedly in my practice is the relationship between patient mindset, trust, and the ultimate success of rhinoplasty. Those who approach their journey with patience, positivity, and trust in both their surgeon and the healing process tend to experience smoother recoveries and better outcomes.

Trusting Your Surgeon and the Process

Your surgeon's experience, eye for beauty, and technical precision are crucial elements in achieving the elegant, natural-looking result you desire. However, even the most skilled surgeon can't deliver an ideal result if their expertise is constantly overridden by excessive patient control. It's completely understandable to have specific goals for your nose, but insisting on controlling every detail—every angle, every millimeter—can do more harm than good.

. . .

In my practice, I often treat executives, models, celebrities, and other high-achieving individuals who are used to calling the shots in their everyday lives. Understandably, that control doesn't just disappear in the consultation room. Yet, rhinoplasty is not something that benefits from micromanagement. Just as you wouldn't hire a world-class architect to design your home and then change every structural detail they recommend, you should avoid dictating every surgical detail. Similarly, walking into a couture atelier and demanding endless adjustments removes the essence of what initially attracted you—the expertise and artistry of the designer. At some point, it ceases to be their creation, becoming something else entirely—and usually, that something else is not ideal.

Of course, it's essential to do your research and carefully choose a surgeon whose expertise, approach, and style resonate with you. Ask questions, review their work, and understand their philosophy. But once you've done this due diligence and made your choice, it's equally important to step back and trust the professional you've selected. Allow them to do their best work. Give yourself permission to relinquish some control and trust the process.

Early in my career, I sometimes gave in to such patient-driven modifications, believing I could seamlessly incorporate them into my approach. However, every time I compromised my judgment, the outcome fell short—not due to technical errors, but because the aesthetic balance was compromised. Today, if I feel strongly that a requested modification will detract from the outcome, I simply won't proceed with it. Trust is foundational. If you chose your surgeon for their expertise, aesthetic judgment, and technical skill, trust them enough to guide you through the process.

. . .

Avoid the Trap of Mirror Obsession

One common challenge I see during rhinoplasty recovery is what I call "mirror obsession." Some patients scrutinize their noses constantly, checking from various angles, lighting conditions, and even taking numerous selfies. This constant scrutiny creates unnecessary stress. The reality is this: no rhinoplasty heals perfectly linearly or symmetrically at every stage. Swelling fluctuates, minor asymmetries may appear temporarily, and subtle variations occur frequently during the healing timeline. This is entirely normal.

Those who embrace the natural ups and downs of healing, avoid excessive manipulation, and trust the body's inherent ability to heal tend to experience smoother recoveries and, ultimately, more satisfying results. Over-cleaning, excessive touching, or constantly questioning the process can actually disrupt delicate healing tissues, leading to prolonged swelling or even less predictable results.

Less is More

Healing from rhinoplasty isn't linear. Swelling fluctuates, and subtle asymmetries will come and go before stabilizing. Patience is crucial. The nose you see at one month isn't your final nose—it continues refining itself, often dramatically, for up to a year after surgery.

Patients who accept that the journey involves some uncertainty, follow their surgeon's instructions diligently without trying to accelerate the process, and resist micromanaging each sensation or visual change invariably do best. The body knows what it's doing—give it the space and time to do so.

. . .

Importance of Follow-Up Care

An essential aspect of successful rhinoplasty recovery is regular follow-up care. You and your surgeon are partners in this journey and trust is key. Occasionally, patients skip follow-up visits, either assuming everything is fine or fearing that something is wrong. This is a critical error. Regular follow-ups aren't just formalities—they're integral checkpoints. Early on, minor issues can usually be addressed easily, preventing complications down the line. Even if you feel fine or worry something is wrong, communicate openly with your surgeon. I cannot emphasize this enough. Trust your surgeon not only during surgery but also through your entire healing journey.

Patience: The Hardest but Most Crucial Ingredient

I often remind my patients: *"The nose you see at one month is not the nose you'll see at six months, and certainly not the nose you'll have at one year."* Rhinoplasty is a long-term journey. Swelling fluctuates, minor asymmetries may come and go, and the final result takes time—often up to a year. Understanding and embracing this process makes all the difference.

For the best outcome, trust your surgeon's expertise rather than fixating on every detail. Resist the urge to scrutinize your nose in the mirror daily; healing is a gradual process, and patience yields the best results. Less intervention, more time, and a steady, natural recovery often lead to the most beautiful and lasting changes. Keep communication open with your surgeon, especially at follow-up visits, to ensure you stay on track.

• • •

Rhinoplasty is an artful collaboration between patient and surgeon. You've chosen your surgeon for their skill, vision, and experience, now, trust that decision. The nose knows how to heal; your role is to give it the space and time to do so.

Trusting the process doesn't mean ignoring your concerns, it means creating the right conditions for success: Open communication, patience, care, and confidence in the journey ahead.

CHAPTER 31
FINAL THOUGHTS

Choosing to undergo rhinoplasty is not just about reshaping your nose—it's about refining your confidence, enhancing your harmony, and making a choice that feels right for you. This is an incredibly personal decision, one that should be made with clarity, self-awareness, and the right guidance.

This book is not about persuading you to have surgery, or not have surgery, or promising a specific outcome. I write this book to empower you with the knowledge to make an informed decision—one rooted in truth, not trends; in self-reflection, not pressure. This is not a manual on surgical techniques or recovery timelines. It is a conversation about understanding your motivations, setting realistic expectations, and approaching your decision for or against having a rhinoplasty with the tools you need to make your right decision.

Before anything else, ask yourself: why do I want this? Your motivation matters more than anything. Are you doing this for yourself, or are external influences shaping your decision? Are you seeking balance and harmony, or chasing an impossible idea of perfection?

While rhinoplasty can have an incredible positive impact on your confidence and breathing, it is not a cure-all for deeper insecurities or emotional struggles. Some patients arrive with filtered selfies, celebrity photos, or digitally altered versions of their own faces, hoping for a dramatic reinvention. But rhinoplasty is not about imitation—it's about elevating what makes you uniquely you.

Just as important as the decision to undergo surgery is the choice of who performs it. Rhinoplasty is one of the most intricate and challenging cosmetic procedures, requiring both technical precision and an artistic eye. A skilled surgeon doesn't just operate, they sculpt, refine, and balance. They understand that no two noses should look the same because no two faces are the same. The best rhinoplasty is one that looks effortless, where the result is so natural that no one can quite tell what has changed, only that your face appears more balanced, harmonious, and right.

The most beautiful noses don't demand attention. They don't overpower. They complement. They refine. They enhance without erasing identity.

More than anything, this journey is about self-awareness. Rhinoplasty should never be a decision made out of insecurity but rather a step taken with intention. Your face tells a story—your story—and any change to it should feel authentic to who you are, not a departure from it. Beauty is not about conforming to a singular ideal; it is about embracing and enhancing what is already yours.

The decision to have surgery is yours and yours alone. Others may have opinions, but ultimately, this is your journey, your face, your choice. If you are reading this book, you have already taken the reins of informed decision-making in your own hands. Whatever you decide, let it be a choice that empowers you. Let it be a decision made with confidence, not doubt. And most importantly, let it be one that aligns with the person you are, the person you aspire to be, the life you aspire to live.

ABOUT THE AUTHOR

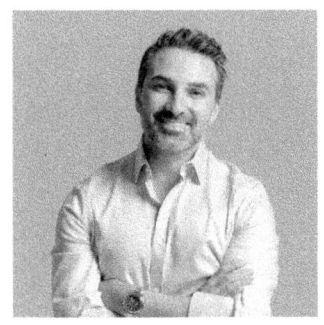

Masoud Saman, MD, FACS is an educator, author, and double board-certified facial plastic surgeon, internationally recognized as a leading authority in rhinoplasty and facial rejuvenation. Before dedicating his career solely to facial aesthetics, he led a busy head and neck cancer center, performing life-saving cancer and reconstructive surgeries.

With over a decade dedicated to facial aesthetics and reconstruction, Dr. Saman has become the surgeon of choice for discerning patients worldwide, including celebrities seeking exceptional results. His signature "*Saman Nose*" seamlessly blends American safety standards with European aesthetic refinement. A relentless perfectionist, he approaches surgery as an art, obsessing over craftsmanship to create the best possible outcome for each patient.

instagram.com/samanplasticsurgery

www.ingramcontent.com/pod-product-compliance
Lightning Source LLC
Chambersburg PA
CBHW052128030426
42337CB00028B/5074